Advance Acclaim For

PSYCHOTROPIC DRUGS AND WOMEN: FAST FACTS

"This welcome handbook is chock-full of practical pearls and other assorted clinical gems. *Psychotropic Drugs and Women* is likely to be the first resource clinicians reach for when seeking consultation on tricky questions concerning the psychopharmacological management of women in all stages of life. Readers will quickly find what they need to know about the use of all contemporary psychiatric medications in women of reproductive age and during pregnancy, nursing, perimenopause, postmenopause, and virtually all situations pertinent to every day practice. This treasure trove of information is presented in a highly readable, easily accessible format."

— Joel Yager, M.D., Professor of Psychiatry,
University of New Mexico School of Medicine

"This easy-to-use handbook provides practical and up-to-date information on the pharmacologic treatment of the most common psychiatric disorders in women, with special consideration given to the effects of gender and reproductive factors on treatment decisions. A great reference for both primary care and specialty clinicians who want to improve their care of women patients."

— Susan G. Kornstein, M.D., Professor of Psychiatry and
Obstetrics/Gynecology, Director, Institute for Women's Health,
Virginia Commonwealth University

D0012345

PSYCHOTROPIC
DRUGS
AND
WOMEN
FAST
FACTS

OTHER BOOKS IN THE FAST FACTS SERIES

Psychotropic Drugs: Fast Facts, Third Edition
by Jerrold S. Maxmen, M.D., Nicholas G. Ward, M.D.
with Steven L. Dubovsky, M.D. as special advisor

Sexual Pharmacology: Fast Facts
by Robert Taylor Segraves, M.D., Ph.D., and Richard Balon, M.D.

Psychotropic Drugs and the Elderly: Fast Facts
by Joel Sadavoy, M.D., FRCP (C)

A NORTON PROFESSIONAL BOOK

PSYCHOTROPIC
DRUGS
AND
WOMEN
FAST
ATS

Victoria Hendrick, M.D.
Michael Gitlin, M.D.

W. W. Norton & Company
New York • London

NOTICE

We have made every attempt to summarize accurately and concisely a number of references. However, the reader is reminded that times and medical knowledge change, transcription or understanding error is always possible, and crucial details are omitted whenever such a comprehensive distillation as this is attempted in limited space. We cannot, therefore, guarantee that every bit of information is absolutely accurate or complete. The reader should affirm that cited recommendations are still appropriate by reading the original articles and checking other sources including local consultants and recent literature.

DRUG DOSAGE
The author and publisher have exerted every effort to ensure that drug selection and dosage set forth in this text are in accord with current recommendations and practice at the time of publication. However, in view of ongoing research, changes in government regulations, and the constant flow of information relating to drug therapy and drug reactions, the reader is urged to check the package insert for each drug for any change in indications and dosage and for added warnings and precautions. This is particularly important when the recommended agent is a new and/or infrequently used drug.

Copyright © 2004 by Victoria Hendrick, M.D., and Michael Gitlin, M.D.

All rights reserved
Printed in the United States of America
First Edition

For information about permission to reproduce
selections from this book, write to
Permissions, W. W. Norton & Company, Inc.,
500 Fifth Avenue, New York, NY 10110

Production Manager: Leeann Graham
Manufactured by Quebecor World Fairfield

Library of Congress Cataloging-in-Publication Data

Hendrick, Victoria C., 1963–
    Psychotropic drugs and women / Victoria Hendrick, Michael Gitlin.
        p. ; cm. — (Fast facts)
    "A Norton professional book."
    Includes bibliographical references and index.
    ISBN 0-393-70421-1
    1. Psychotropic drugs. 2. Women—Mental health.   3. Mental illness—
    Chemotherapy. I. Gitlin, Michael J. II. Title. III. Fast facts
    (New York, N.Y.)
    [DNLM: 1. Psychotropic Drugs—contraindications.   2. Mental Disorders—
    drug therapy.   3. Sex Factors.   4. Women's Health. QV 77.2 H498p 2004]
    RM315.H46 2004
    615′.788—dc22   2003061408

W. W. Norton & Company, Inc., 500 Fifth Avenue, New York, N.Y. 10110
www.wwnorton.com

W. W. Norton & Company Ltd., Castle House, 75/76 Wells St., London W1T 3QT

1 3 5 7 9 0 8 6 4 2

DEDICATIONS

To Tobias, whose enthusiasm and curiosity inspire me to broaden my own learning, and to Alex, whose love and support give me the strength to take on new challenges.
—V. H.

To my three children:
Katie and Rebecca, who exemplify the intelligent, informed women of the next generation, and Josh, who is more respectful of women than any man I know.
—M. G.

Contents

C O N T E N T S

CONTENTS

Abbreviations

ACE	angiotensin-converting enzyme		FDA	Food and Drug Administration, United States
AEDs	antiepileptic drugs		FSH	follicle-stimulating hormone
AIDS	acquired immunodeficiency syndrome			
			GABA	gamma-aminobutyric acid
			GAD	generalized anxiety disorder
β-HCG	β-human chorionic gonadotropin		GI	gastrointenstinal
			GnRH	gonadotropin releasing hormone
BED	binge eating disorder			
Bid	twice a day			
BMI	body mass index		HCG	human chorionic gonadotropin
CBC	complete blood count		HDL	high-density lipoprotein
CNS	central nervous system		HDRS	Hamilton Depression Rating Scale
CPK	creatinine kinase			
CR	controlled release		HIV	human immunodeficiency virus
CRH	corticotropin releasing hormone		HRT	hormone replacement therapy
CYP	cytochrome			
DES	diethylstilbestrol		IM	intramuscular
DHA	docosahexanoic acid		IR	immediate release
DHEA	dehydroepiandrosterone		IVF	in vitro fertilization
DHEAS	dehydroepiandrosterone sulfate		LH	luteinizing hormone
DM	dextromethorphan			
DSM	*Diagnostic and Statistical Maual*		MAO	monoamine oxidase
			MAOIs	monoamine oxidase inhibitors
ECT	electroconvulsive therapy		mCPP	m-chlorophenylpiperazine
EKG	electrocardiogram		MRI	magnetic resonance imaging
EPA	eicosapentaenoic acid			
EPS	extrapyramidal symptoms		NCS	National Comorbidity Survey
ER	extended release		NIH	National Institutes of Health, United States
ERT	estrogen replacement therapy			

NMS	neuroleptic malignant syndrome	QT	QT interval on EKG
NSAIDs	non-steroidal anti-inflammatory drugs	QTc	corrected QT interval on EKG
NTDs	neural tube defects	RIMAs	reversible monoamine oxidase inhibitors
OCs	oral contraceptives		
OCD	obsessive-compulsive disorder	SAD	social anxiety disorder
OTC	over the counter	SNRIs	serotonin norepinephrine reuptake inhibitors
		SR	sustained release
PCOS	polycystic ovary syndrome	SSRIs	selective serotonin reuptake inhibitors
PDR	*Physicians' Desk Reference*		
PMDD	premenstrual dysphoric disorder	TCAs	tricyclic antidepressants
		TD	tardive dyskinesia
PMS	premenstrual syndrome	Tid	three times a day
PTSD	posttraumatic stress disorder	TIS	Teratogen Information Services
		TSH	thyroid stimulating hormone
Q	every		
qid	four times daily	XR	extended release

Preface

When women take psychotropic drugs, their treatment needs are often distinct from those of men. Gender differences emerge in response to treatment, medication side effects, drug interactions, and risk considerations. Some gender considerations are well-recognized, such as the potential risks of medication exposure during pregnancy. Other gender considerations are more subtle and may be overlooked in the course of clinical practice.

This book provides information for the treatment of psychiatric disorders across women's reproductive lives. Besides reviewing female-specific considerations, each chapter provides information necessary for the general psychopharmacologic treatment of women presenting with psychiatric conditions. Subsections of each chapter review the treatment of psychiatric disorders at different life stages, including reproductive years, pregnancy, breast-feeding, peri-menopause, and post-menopause. Female endocrinology and gender differences in drug metabolism are also reviewed.

Psychotropic Drugs and Women: Fast Facts is organized around the treatment of the principal psychiatric diagnoses: depressive disorders, bipolar disorder, anxiety disorders, and schizophrenia. For medications that are used to treat more than one psychiatric disorder, details on their use are listed under the psychiatric disorder for which they are primarily prescribed (e.g., benzodiazepines for generalized anxiety disorder).

The focus on pharmacologic treatment should not detract from the use of psychotherapeutic approaches. These approaches are particularly essential for certain conditions—e.g., eating disorders and posttraumatic stress disorder—for which psychotherapy, not medication, is typically the primary treatment. For all patients, multifaceted approaches that include pharmacotherapy, psychotherapy, and attention to psychosocial stressors are most likely to be successful.

Victoria Hendrick, M.D.
Michael Gitlin, M.D.

Acknowledgments

This book was inspired by our work with patients, residents and colleagues at UCLA's Neuropsychiatric Hospital. Our patients have helped us understand how gender often influences the course of treatment and must not be overlooked in clinical practice. The psychiatry residents of UCLA, who keep us on our toes with their sharp and inquisitive questions, continuously stimulate us to hone our clinical practices and teaching skills. Finally, we are fortunate to work with colleagues whose knowledge and curiosity keep our intellectual lives rich and growing. We are particularly indebted to Drs. Carole Edelstein, Andrea Rapkin, Wendy Rosenstein, Michael Smith, and Deborah Yaeger, who read and provided thoughtful feedback on several sections of the book, and to Drs. Lori Altshuler, Vivien Burt, Kathleen Daly, Mark Frye, and Rita Suri for their daily presence in our mutual clinical, teaching, and research endeavors.

A
C
K
N
O
W
L
E
D
G
M
E
N
T
S

PSYCHOTROPIC
DRUGS
AND
WOMEN
FAST
FACTS

1. General Considerations in the Psychopharmacological Treatment of Women

INTRODUCTION

The effective and safe use of psychotropic medications in women requires an awareness of gender-specific considerations in psychopharmacology. For many years, women's health care was compromised by a lack of information on gender differences. Following the thalidomide tragedy of the late 1950s and the abnormalities identified in children of pregnant women exposed to diethylstilbestrol (DES), the Food and Drug Administration (FDA) prohibited women of reproductive age from participating in clinical trials.

This policy changed with the National Institute of Health Revitalization Act of 1993, which mandated that women and members of minorities must be included in all research involving human subjects. The FDA, in effect, reversed its prior policy by encouraging the inclusion of women in clinical trials and emphasizing the need for studies examining the impact of gender on the efficacy, metabolism, and side effects of psychotropic medications. Since that time, the literature on these gender-specific considerations has grown steadily.

Nevertheless, many limitations remain in the literature. Gender-based data analyses are still not routinely included in research publications. Consequently, little is known about gender differences in the dosing, efficacy, and metabolism of many medications. The impact of different

3

stages of the menstrual cycle and of the female life cycle (e.g., pre- vs. postmenopausal) on medication metabolism and efficacy also remains to be researched. Psychiatric side effects of medications that are taken primarily or exclusively by women (e.g., ovulation-inducing agents), remain largely unknown.

Further research on the role of gender in treatment is particularly important for women, given that they comprise the majority of patients seeking mental health care and receiving prescriptions for antidepressant and antianxiety medications. With the recent increase in direct-to-consumer advertising, the need for female-specific medication information has become more pressing. Psychiatric medications—mostly antidepressants and anxiolytics—are intensively marketed to women through advertising in magazines, television, and other venues. Not surprisingly, direct-to-consumer advertising has led to an increase in the number of women requesting prescription drugs from their doctors.

An essential consideration in providing pharmacological treatment to women of reproductive age is the possibility of pregnancy. Over 50% of pregnancies in United States are unplanned, and many women become pregnant while taking medications. The psychiatric care of women of reproductive age should routinely include questions about patients' methods of contraception and regularity of use, history of unprotected intercourse, and recent missed menstrual periods. These questions are particularly important for chronically mentally ill women, who are less likely than other women to use regular contraception. Adequate contraception has become particularly important following the widespread use of newer antipsychotic agents that, unlike the older medications, do not interfere with women's ability to conceive.

As women age, their psychopharmacological treatment may need adjusting. Elderly women are generally more vulnerable to medication side effects than their younger counterparts. Furthermore, they are more likely to take multiple medications and therefore face a greater risk for drug–drug interactions and additive medication effects (e.g., sedation). Most psychiatric research has focused on relatively young and healthy populations; therefore, much remains to be learned about the psychopharmacological treatment of elderly women. In working with this population, it is important to keep in mind its heterogeneity: Treatment considerations for a robust 68-year-old woman will most likely differ from those of a frail 85-year-old.

Table 1.1. Lifetime and 12-Month Prevalence Rates of Psychiatric Disorders in Women and Men

	Male		Female		Total	
	Lifetime	12-month	Lifetime	12-month	Lifetime	12-month
Affective Disorders						
Major depressive episode	12.7	7.7	21.3	12.9	17.1	10.3
Manic episode	1.6	1.4	1.7	1.3	1.6	1.3
Dysthymia	4.8	2.1	8.0	3.0	6.4	2.5
Any affective disorder	14.7	8.5	23.9	14.1	19.3	11.3
Anxiety Disorders						
Panic disorder	2.0	1.3	5.0	3.2	3.5	2.3
Agoraphobia w/o panic disorder	3.5	1.7	7.0	3.8	5.3	2.8
Social phobia	11.1	6.6	15.5	9.1	13.3	7.9
Simple phobia	6.7	4.4	15.7	13.2	11.3	8.8
Generalized anxiety disorder	3.6	2.0	6.6	4.3	5.1	3.1
Any anxiety disorder	19.2	11.8	30.5	22.6	24.9	17.2
Substance Use Disorders						
Alcohol abuse w/o dependence	12.5	3.4	6.4	1.6	9.4	2.5
Alcohol dependence	20.1	10.7	8.2	3.7	14.1	7.2
Drug abuse w/o dependence	5.4	1.3	3.5	0.3	4.4	0.8
Drug dependence	9.2	3.8	5.9	1.9	7.5	2.8
Any substance abuse/dependence	35.4	16.1	17.9	6.6	26.6	11.3
Other Disorders						
Antisocial personality	5.8	—	—	—	3.5	—
Nonaffective psychosis[†]	0.3	0.5	0.8	0.6	0.7	0.5
*Any NCS disorder	48.7	27.7	47.3	31.2	48.0	29.5

[†] Nonaffective psychosis includes schizophrenia, schizophreniform disorder, delusional disorder, and atypical psychosis.
* NCS, National Comorbidity Survey.
(*Source:* Kessler RC, McGonagle KA, Zhao S, et al. Lifetime and 12-month prevalence of *DSM-III-R* psychiatric disorders in the United States. Results from the National Comorbidity Survey. *Arch Gen Psychiatry.* 1994; 51[1]: 8–19.)

In providing psychopharmacological medications to women, clinicians should always take into account the psychosocial factors that may contribute to psychiatric symptoms in women. The multiple demands placed on women—to fulfill roles as caregivers of children and, often, aging parents, to earn income, to attend to household duties—often produce considerable stress. Women's vulnerability to domestic and sexual violence is a significant additional stressor.

Elderly women often live alone and may face financial hardship. By listening to and helping women cope with the stresses in their lives, clinicians can minimize their need to use medications. Taking such an approach is particularly important for women who are pregnant or nursing because psychiatric medications readily cross the placenta and enter breast milk.

This book reviews important considerations for clinicians who prescribe psychotropic agents to women. Because treatment considerations may vary at different stages in women's lives, information is provided for each reproductive phase. The book also includes general (i.e., not gender-specific) reviews of the pharmacological management of psychiatric disorders, as this information is clearly relevant to the treatment of female patients.

THE USE OF PSYCHIATRIC MEDICATIONS FOR WOMEN OF ALL AGES

* Evaluate women for symptoms of thyroid dysfunction.
    √ Women are at greater risk of thyroid dysfunction (hyper- or hypothyroidism) than men.
    √ Symptoms of thyroid dysfunction are listed in Table 1.2.
* Obtain baseline assessments of patients' sexual functioning before beginning medications.
    √ Many psychiatric medications can cause sexual dysfunction (e.g., anorgasmia, reduced libido).
    √ Assessments of sexual functioning should continue over the course of treatment, particularly after any changes in medications or dosage.

Table 1.2. Symptoms of Thyroid Dysfunction

Symptoms of Hyperthyroidism	Symptoms of Hypothyroidism
Anxiety	Poor concentration
Insomnia	Dry hair and skin; hair loss
Weight loss	Weight gain
Tachycardia	Bradycardia
Shortness of breath	Myxedemic or puffy appearance
Fatigue	Fatigue
Heat intolerance	Cold intolerance
Muscle weakness	Muscle cramps
Tremor	Constipation
Menstrual irregularity	Menstrual irregularity

* Before initiating a new medication, discuss its potential impact on appetite and weight; many women will not be willing to take medications that produce weight gain.
* Consider obtaining weight measurements if a patient is on a medication that may produce weight gain (e.g., lithium, valproate, olanzapine).
  √ One approach is to calculate BMI (body mass index: weight in kg divided by height in meters squared):
    □ BMI of 25–29.9: overweight.
    □ BMI of 30 or more: obesity.

* Ask about use of medications that may produce mood changes, including:
  √ GnRH agonists (e.g., leuprolide [Lupron], nafarelin [Synarel], goserelin [Zoladex]—used for endometriosis, uterine fibroids, IVF).
  √ Hormonal contraception (see Chapter 9).
  √ Antihypertensive agents (e.g., beta-blockers, angiotensin-converting enzyme [ACE] inhibitors, calcium channel blockers).
  √ Lipid-lowering agents.

GENERAL CONSIDERATIONS

THE USE OF PSYCHIATRIC MEDICATIONS IN WOMEN OF REPRODUCTIVE AGE

* Document patients' menstrual pattern before and after initiating psychiatric medications.
* Menstrual cycles can be monitored with a chart such as the one shown in Figure 7.1.
  √ Normal menstrual cycle length is between 22 and 35 days.
  √ Menstrual cycle abnormalities:
    □ Amenorrhea: No menstruation for three or more cycles.
    □ Oligomenorrhea: Cycle length longer than 35 days.
    □ Irregular menstrual cycle: Cycle length varying more than 4 days from cycle to cycle.
  √ Hyperprolactinemia is a potential side effect of several antidepressant and antipsychotic medications (see Chapters 3 and 6).
  √ Elevated prolactin inhibits the hypothalamic–pituitary–ovarian axis and can produce menstrual irregularities or amenorrhea.

√ Prolactin secretion is normally inhibited by dopamine; if dopamine level diminishes (as with antipsychotic agents), prolactin level rises.

√ Prolactin level also rises with an increase in serotonergic activity.

• In the work-up of menstrual irregularities and amenorrhea, include:

√ Prolactin level (normal level for women of reproductive age: 5–29 ng/ml).

√ Pregnancy test: β-human chorionic gonadotropin (β-HCG).

√ Thyroid panel (hypothyroidism can produce menstrual irregularities).

√ If there is evidence of polycystic ovary syndrome (e.g., irregular menses, hirsutism, acne, obesity), obtain androgen levels (serum testosterone and androstenedione).

• Evaluate for premenstrual exacerbation of symptoms.

√ Depression, bipolar disorder, anxiety, and psychosis can worsen premenstrually.

√ If patient experiences a recurrent premenstrual relapse or exacerbation of psychiatric symptoms, consider increasing medication dose by 50% at midcycle.

Contraception and Family Planning

• Advise sexually active heterosexual women who do not wish to conceive to use an effective method of contraception.

• Consider the potential impact of concomitant medications on hormonal contraception.

√ Hormonal contraceptives can be rendered ineffective by the concomitant use of medications that increase their metabolism, including:

▫ Carbamazepine.

▫ Oxcarbazepine.

▫ Topiramate.

▫ Modafinil.

▫ St. John's wort.

√ Women should be encouraged to use a high-potency oral contraceptive (i.e., containing at least 50 μg/day of estradiol) or an alternative method of contraception while taking these medications.

- Consider the potential impact of hormonal contraceptives on concomitant medications.
  - √ Estrogen-containing hormonal contraceptives inhibit CYP3A4 (a cytochrome P450 enzyme involved in the metabolism of multiple medications).
    - □ Reported to reduce medication clearance by 40–84% for diazepam, chlordiazepoxide, and imipramine.
    - □ Additional medications that are oxidatively metabolized by CYP3A4 are listed in Chapter 2.
  - √ Estrogen-containing hormonal contraceptives can induce hepatic conjugative enzymes and may therefore increase the metabolism of medications that are conjugated before elimination by the kidney.
    - □ Reported to alter lamotrigine levels by 40–60% in one small case series.
- Inquire about patients' plans regarding pregnancy.
  - √ For women planning to conceive in near future, attempt to prescribe medications for which safety data exist during pregnancy (see the next section).
- Obtain a pregnancy test before initiating or continuing psychiatric medications in women who have recently had unprotected intercourse or have missed their menstrual period.
  - √ An over-the-counter (OTC) pregnancy test can be used that
    - □ Registers positive 12–14 days after conception.
    - □ Is simple to use.
    - □ Provides results within 5–10 minutes.
    - □ Is 98% accurate.
  - √ Alternatively, obtain a blood test for β-human chorionic gonadotropin (β-HCG); this is 99–100% accurate.
- Regardless of methods of contraception used, encourage the use of condoms to reduce the risk of HIV transmission.
  - √ Especially important for chronically mentally ill women, who are at increased risk for AIDS compared to women without mental illness.

GENERAL PRINCIPLES FOR USE OF PSYCHOTROPIC MEDICATIONS DURING PREGNANCY

- Whenever possible, review treatment options in pregnancy prior to a woman's discontinuation of contraception.

- If a patient is likely to remain psychiatrically stable, even without medications, for several weeks or longer, consider tapering and discontinuing the medication before she attempts to conceive.
  - √ This approach is particularly reasonable for women who are likely to conceive quickly (i.e., healthy, < 35 years old, with no history of infertility in themselves or their partners).
  - √ Educate patients about ways to maximize chances of conception as quickly as possible by using methods to detect ovulation.
    - □ By monitoring basal body temperature or using an OTC ovulation detection kit.
- Alternatively, the medication can be discontinued as late as the second gestational week, when a pregnancy test turns positive. This approach is reasonable for women who are *not* likely to conceive quickly. Once the pregnancy test is positive, and patient remains stable, discontinue the medication.
  - √ The uteroplacental circulation forms at approximately 2 weeks postconception.
  - √ Therefore, the embryo receives minimal exposure.
- Certain medications should be tapered rather than stopped abruptly to avoid withdrawal symptoms and reduce likelihood of relapse (e.g., paroxetine, venlafaxine, lithium; see Chapters 3 and 4).
- Certain medications should be used only if absolutely necessary in the first trimester, particularly the first 6 weeks postconception.
  - √ Valproate and carbamazepine are linked with a substantial risk of neural tube defects when used in first 6 weeks of pregnancy (see Chapter 4).
- When medications are used in pregnancy, maintain the lowest dosage and fewest medications necessary for control of symptoms.
- Whenever possible, try to postpone use of medications until after 12th gestational week:
  - √ Particularly important for medications with limited safety data in pregnancy.
- Gestational age is determined from the date of a woman's last menstrual period, *not* from the date of conception.
  - √ Conception typically occurs approximately 2 weeks after a menstrual period.
  - √ Therefore, the actual fetal age is about 2 weeks less than the gestational age.

Table 1.3. Risk–Benefit Discussion of Psychiatric Treatment During Pregnancy

G
E
N
E
R
A
L

C
O
N
S
I
D
E
R
A
T
I
O
N
S

- Discuss available data on exposures to the psychiatric medication during pregnancy and lactation.
- Review patient's likelihood of a psychiatric relapse during pregnancy and the postpartum period.
- Review measures that may reduce likelihood of relapse (e.g., psychotherapy; couples counseling; change in work schedule; assistance with child care responsibilities).
- Whenever the patient allows, include baby's father, health-care professionals (obstetrician, midwife, pediatrician, lactation consultant) in the risk–benefit discussion.
- Inform patients about the limitations of current research findings, including:
  √ Small sample sizes.
  √ Limited information on potential neurobehavioral sequelae of prenatal medication exposure.
  √ Lack of control, in most studies, for maternal health habits and concomitant use of medications and substances such as nicotine, alcohol.
- Inform patients that approximately 2–4% of infants are born with birth defects, regardless of prenatal medication exposure.
- Include a statement indicating that the patient has been told and understands the benefits and risks involved in the decision and is in agreement with the treatment plan.
- Document the risk–benefit discussion in the patient's file.
- Continue to document ongoing risk–benefit analyses over the course of the pregnancy.

√ The 12th gestational week corresponds to a fetal age of approximately 10 weeks.

- Medication doses may require adjustment during pregnancy because of increased liver metabolism, decreased protein binding, and greater volume of distribution (see Chapter 2).
- Emphasize importance of avoiding nicotine, alcohol, and all illicit drugs during the pregnancy.
- Perform and record a careful risk–benefit discussion of treatment considerations (Table 1.3).
- Research data primarily come from:
  √ Naturalistic studies.
  √ Reports of pregnancy outcomes from callers to Teratogen Information Services (TIS).
  √ Single case reports or small case series.
  √ Pharmaceutical company pregnancy registries.

Nicotine Use During Pregnancy

- Smoking during pregnancy is linked with increased risk of miscarriage, low birth weight, perinatal mortality, and attention-deficit disorder in children.
- Risk is directly related to number of cigarettes/day:
  < 1 pack of cigarettes/day: Risk of low birth-weight infant increases by 50% above baseline.
  > 1 pack/day: Risk increases by 130%.

Table 1.4. Food and Drug Administration Use-in-Pregnancy Ratings

A	Controlled studies in women show no risk.
B	Animal studies show no risk, but there are no controlled studies in humans; or animal studies show adverse effect that has not been confirmed in human studies.
C	Animal studies show risk, but there are no controlled studies in humans; or studies in animals and humans are not available.
D	There is evidence of risk in humans, but the drug may have benefits that outweigh the risk.
X	Risk outweighs any benefit.

Source: (Key to FDA Use-in-Pregnancy ratings. In *Physicians' Desk Reference*, 55th Edition. Montvale, NJ: Medical Economics Company, 2001; p. 344.)

- If the mother quits smoking by 16 weeks of pregnancy, risk to fetus is similar to that of a nonsmoking mother.
- Strongly urge patients to stop or reduce smoking!
- If necessary, refer patients to behavioral techniques, support groups.
- Prescribe nicotine patches or gum while patient is trying to conceive.
  √ Not recommended for use during pregnancy.
- Prescribe bupropion (Wellbutrin, Zyban; see pp. 45–47).
  √ Can be used during pregnancy to help reduce nicotine use.

Alcohol Use During Pregnancy

- Use of alcohol during pregnancy can cause mental retardation, malformation, growth retardation, miscarriage, and behavioral disorders in infants.
- As with nicotine, the adverse effects are dose related:
  √ 11% of infants affected if mother consumes two to four drinks/day.
  √ 19% of infants affected if mother consumes > four drinks/day.
- If necessary, refer patients to an alcohol rehabilitation program.

Illicit Drug Use During Pregnancy

- Heroin use during pregnancy is associated with intrauterine growth restriction, hyperactivity, and neonatal withdrawal.
- Cocaine use during pregnancy is associated with miscarriage, prematurity, growth retardation, and congenital defects.

Table 1.5. Food and Drug Administration Use-in-Pregnancy Ratings for Specific Medications

Medication	FDA Use-in-Pregnancy Rating
Anxiolytics and Sedatives	
alprazolam (Xanax)	D
buspirone (Buspar)	B
clonazepam (Klonopin)	D
diazepam (Valium)	D
flurazepam (Dalmane)	X
lorazepam (Ativan)	D
temazepam (Restoril)	X
zolpidem (Ambien)	B
Antidepressants	
amitriptyline (Elavil, Endep)	D
bupropion (Wellbutrin)	B
citalopram (Celexa, Lexapro)	C
clomipramine (Anafranil)	C
desipramine (Norpramin, Pertofrane)	C
doxepin (Adapin, Sinequan)	C
fluoxetine (Prozac, Sarafem)	C
fluvoxamine (Luvox)	C
imipramine (Tofranil)	D
mirtazapine (Hemeron)	C
nefazodone (Serzone)	C
nortriptyline (Aventyl, Pamelor)	D
paroxetine (Paxil)	C
sertraline (Zoloft)	C
trazodone (Desyrel)	C
venlafaxine (Effexor)	C
Mood Stabilizers	
lithium (Lithobid, Eskalith)	D
valproate (Depakote, Depakene)	D
carbamazepine (Tegretol)	D
gabapentin (Neurontin)	C
lamotrigine (Lamictal)	C
oxcarbazepine (Trileptal)	C
Antipsychotics	
aripiprazole (Abilify)	C
clozapine (Clozaril)	B
fluphenazine (Prolixin)	C
haloperidol (Haldol)	C
olanzapine (Zyprexa)	C
risperidone (Risperdal)	C
quetiapine (Seroquel)	C
trifluoperazine (Stelazine)	C
ziprasidone (Geodon)	C
Stimulants	
dextroamphetamine (Adderall, Dexedrine)	C
methylphenidate (Ritalin)	C
modafinil (Provigil)	C
Anticholinergic Agents	
diphenhydramine (Benadryl)	B
hydroxyzine (Atarax)	C
trihexyphenidyl (Artane)	C

(cont.)

GENERAL CONSIDERATIONS

Table 1.5. *Continued*

Medication	FDA Use-in-Pregnancy Rating
Antihypertensive Agents	
propanolol (Inderal)	C
clonidine (Catapres)	C
Hormone Supplements	
levothyroxine (Synthroid)	A
oral contraceptives	X
Analgesics	
acetaminophen (Tylenol)	B
ibuprofen (Motrin)	B
naproxen (Naprosyn)	B
sumatriptan (Imitrex)	C

- If necessary, refer patients to substance abuse treatment programs, ideally to be completed before conception.
- Periodic urine drug testing may help to encourage abstinence.
- A methadone maintenance program during pregnancy is preferable to continued use of heroin.

Food and Drug Administration Labeling for Medications

- Medications carrying an FDA Pregnancy Category B rating are not necessarily safer to use in pregnancy than medications with Pregnancy Category C labeling.
- Medications for which no human data exist may receive the Category B rating if animal studies have not found a fetal risk.
- Category C-labeled medications for which human data show low risk may be preferable to Category B-labeled medications for which there are no human data.

GENERAL PRINCIPLES FOR USE OF PSYCHOTROPIC MEDICATIONS DURING BREAST-FEEDING

- Infants' ability to metabolize medications increases from approximately 33% of adult (weight-adjusted) capacity at birth to 100% at 6 months of age.
- Therefore, exposure to medications through breast milk may be riskier for newborns than for older infants.
- Whenever possible, choose medications for which safety data exist on their use in breast-feeding.

- Prescribe the minimum dosage of medication that produces remission of mother's symptoms.
- Consider supplementation with bottle feeding to reduce the infant's exposure to medications through breast milk.

Serum Concentrations of Medication in Nursing Infants

- Infant serum concentrations provide a measure of infant's exposure to medication through breast milk.
- However, the blood draw can be traumatic to the infant, and the information is of limited value.
  - √ No cutoff has been established for a safe serum level of medication in infants.
- Serum levels need not be obtained routinely in a nursing infant. However, data may provide reassurance for some mothers, especially if the concentration is very low or undetectable.
- To obtain an infant serum concentration of medication:
  - √ Wait until medication serum levels are likely to be at steady state (i.e., at least five medication half-lives).
  - √ Ask the laboratory to use a high-sensitivity assay (i.e., with a limit of detection < 2 ng/ml).
  - √ Measure concentrations of both the parent drug and its metabolites in infant serum.

Additional Issues for Nursing Mothers of Adopted or Premature Infants

- Certain medications potently stimulate prolactin release and therefore may produce galactorrhea (nipple discharge), including:
  - √ Metoclopramide (Reglan) and domperidone (Motilium) primarily used to treat nausea, heartburn, and gastroesophageal reflux.
  - √ Sometimes used by nursing women to increase breast milk production.
- Metoclopramide:
  - √ Side effects include nervousness, irritability, depression, and sedation.
  - √ Nursing infants' estimated intake is approximately at 1–5% of the recommended therapeutic dose for children (0.5 mg/kg/day; metoclopramide is used to treat gastroesophageal reflux in infants).
  - √ Because of metoclopramide's side effects, many mothers do not like to use it and have turned instead to domperidone.

Table 1.6. Factors Influencing Infant's Exposure to Medication Through Breast Milk

Maternal Dose

• Medications should be maintained at the lowest effective dose to minimize infant's exposure.

Timing of Maternal Dose

• Concentrations of some drugs are known to peak a few hours after maternal ingestion of the medication.
  √ Sertraline and fluoxetine levels are highest 6–10 hours after mother takes the medication.
  √ By pumping and discarding milk during these hours, mothers can reduce infants' medication exposure.
• However, the time when medications peak in breast milk is unknown for most medications.

Medication Properties

• Half-life: Shorter half-life produces less exposure.
• Protein-binding: Higher protein-binding produces less exposure.
• Potency: Medications vary widely in their potency.
  √ Fluoxetine has approximately one-sixth and one-fifteenth the serotonergic potency of sertraline and paroxetine, respectively.
  √ Therefore, a serum concentration of 100 ng/ml of fluoxetine is approximately equivalent in potency to a serum concentration of 6.7 ng/ml of paroxetine.

- Domperidone:
  √ Has fewer side effects because it does not enter the brain tissue in significant amounts.
  √ However, is not approved for use in the United States.
  √ Nevertheless, women have obtained it by ordering it from pharmacies outside the United States.
  √ It is used particularly by mothers with little or no milk supply (e.g., mothers of a premature or adopted infant).
  √ Highly protein bound (93%) with short half-life, and therefore is not likely to accumulate in breast milk, but the amount of exposure to the nursing infant has not been established.

Mental Illness and Parenting

- Mental illnesses, particularly if severe and chronic, can significantly impair parenting abilities.
- Several psychiatric medications may adversely affect parenting by producing excessive sedation or a flattened affect.
- Important parenting domains to be explored in individuals with mental illness are listed in Table 1.7.
- It is important to distinguish between chronic parenting deficits and deficits that emerge only during times of relapse of a psychiatric condition (e.g., a manic episode).

Table 1.7. Parenting Domains to be Explored in Individuals With Mental Illness

Patient's Mental Status	Patient's Parenting Capacities
Level of disturbance, instability, or violent tendencies (impulse control)	Capacity to attend to child's physical, social and emotional needs
Level of paranoia	Capacity to provide a stable and nurturing environment
Alcohol and drug addiction	Age-appropriate understanding and expectations of child
Compliance with treatment recommendations	Capacity to initiate or follow and enjoy child-centered activity No evidence of physical or sexual abuse Sense of responsibility for self, child and family Capacity to acknowledge any risk to child Capacity to form trusting relationships
Child's Status	**Partner/Spouse's Involvement**
Child's developmental progress	Attitude of partner/spouse toward partner's illness
Child's attachment to parent	Relationship of partner/spouse to child Commitment of partner/spouse to maintaining the family Capacity of partner/spouse to intervene on child's behalf, if and when necessary History of domestic violence

Source: (Adapted from Gopfert M, Webster J, Pollard Nelki. *Parental Psychiatric Disorder: Distressed Parents and Their Families.* Cambridge U.K.: Cambridge University Press; 1996.)

- Clinicians should encourage patients, especially those with young children, to identify family members or friends who can help with child-care responsibilities during future relapses of the illness.
- If chronic parenting deficits are identified, consider making a referral to a parenting education class.

THE USE OF PSYCHIATRIC MEDICATIONS FOR PERI- AND POSTMENOPAUSAL WOMEN

- Evaluate for occurrence of vasomotor symptoms (e.g., hot flashes, night sweats).
  √ These produce symptoms that may be misdiagnosed as anxiety attacks (e.g., flushing, palpitations, shortness of breath).
  √ Follicle-stimulating hormone (FSH) and estradiol levels are helpful in identifying perimenopausal and menopausal status.

GENERAL CONSIDERATIONS

√ FSH level should be obtained on day 2 or 3 of menses.
√ If the level is > 25 mIU/ml, the patient is probably perimenopausal.
√ If the level is > 40 mIU/ml and menstrual cycles have ceased,
the patient is menopausal.
- Evaluate for thyroid dysfunction (see Table 1.2).
√ Peri- and postmenopausal women are at significantly greater
risk for thyroid dysfunction compared to premenopausal women and men.
- Consider drug–drug interactions between estrogen replacement
therapy and other medications (see Chapter 2, pp 25–29).

THE USE OF PSYCHIATRIC MEDICATIONS FOR ELDERLY WOMEN

- Psychiatric diagnoses (e.g., depression and anxiety disorders)
are frequently overlooked in elderly women because health
professionals often focus more on patients' medical and physical impairments.
- Specific recommendations for the psychopharmacological treatment of elderly patients are frequently lacking. This is particularly true for elderly patients with comorbid medical conditions.
Most psychopharmacological research has focused on younger
(< 65 years), healthier populations.
- Aging is generally associated with several physiological changes,
including:
√ Decreased level of serum albumin, resulting in increased concentrations of unbound (i.e., active) medication.
√ Reduced hepatic blood flow and metabolism.
√ Reduced renal clearance.
- These changes may result in increased serum concentrations and
half-lives of medications, and consequently increased likelihood
of side effects.
√ Medication doses should therefore generally begin at half the
doses used for younger adults.
- Elderly women are frequently on multiple medications.
√ Drug–drug interactions (see Table 2.5) may occur when pa-
tients are on two or more medications.

√ Additive effects may occur from medications that produce similar side effects, such as sedation or anticholinergic effects.

√ Many medications that are used for common medical problems (e.g., hypertension, arthritis, respiratory infections) produce these side effects, as do several psychiatric medications.

• Treatment noncompliance is a particular challenge in the treatment of elderly patients; they may forget when to take their medication or confuse one medication with another.

GENERAL CONSIDERATIONS

2. Gender Differences in Psychopharmacology

As noted in Chapter 1, for many years women of childbearing age were routinely excluded from drug trials due to concern about potential fetal risk because of exposure to a medication. This policy excluded even women who were not sexually active, who reliably used contraception, or whose partners had undergone vasectomies. As a result of this ruling, essential information about safety, efficacy, dosing, and uses of new medications was established solely from data obtained on men. This practice changed in 1993 when the National Institute of Health passed the Revitalization Act, which mandated that women and members of minorities must be included in research involving human subjects.

Although clinical drug trials now routinely include women, the study results are frequently grouped together with those from men—that is, without separate gender-based data analyses. The assumption is made that women and men metabolize medications in the same way. However, a growing literature shows that many medications are metabolized differently by men and women. Reasons for these gender differences include differences in body composition, gastrointestinal transit time, and hepatic clearance (Table 2.1). Additionally, gender differences occur as a result of female-specific conditions, including the menstrual cycle, pregnancy, menopause, and the use of hormonal supplementation (e.g., hormonal contraception, hormone replacement).

GENDER DIFFERENCES

The clinical significance of gender differences in drug metabolism remains to be determined. These differences may account for disparities in the incidence of adverse drug reactions across genders. The significance of these disparities is likely to be highest for drugs with narrow therapeutic ranges. Clearly, additional research is necessary to better delineate these gender differences and their clinical implications.

GENDER DIFFERENCES IN PHARMACOKINETICS OF MEDICATIONS

* Factors that may produce gender differences in the pharmacokinetics of medications are listed in Table 2.1.
* The clinical significance of these factors is unclear.

Table 2.1. Factors That May Produce Gender Differences in Pharmacokinetics

Factor	Gender Difference	Potential Effect on Pharmacokinetics
Body composition	Women have greater percentage of body fat	Greater storage of lipid-soluble medications in adipose tissue can lead to prolonged half-lives of medications in women
Gastrointestinal transit time	Progesterone slows gastrointestinal transit time	The rate at which medications travel through the gastrointestinal system may be longer in women during high-progesterone phases (e.g., premenstrually; during pregnancy), with subsequent greater degree of medication absorption
Gastric acid secretion	Women secrete less gastric acid than men	Women may absorb psychotropic drugs more readily because they are weakly basic
Hepatic metabolism	Gender differences have been identified in certain enzymes (see text) Hepatic metabolism generally increases during pregnancy	Gender differences may occur in clearance rate, dosage requirements, and side effects of medications
Renal clearance	Increases during pregnancy	Gender differences may occur in clearance rate, dosage requirements, and side effects of medications
Drug interactions	The use of some medications (e.g., oral contraceptives) is different in men and women	Gender differences may occur in clearance rate, dosage requirements, and side effects of medications

Table 2.2. Gender Differences in Clearance of Certain Medications

Medication	$F > M$	$F < M$	$F = M$
acetaminophen		X	
alprazolam	X		X*
chlordiazepoxide		X	
clozapine		X	
desipramine		X	
diazepam	X		X*
digoxin		X	
erythromycin	X		
lorazepam			X
naproxen		X	
oxazepam		X	
propanolol		X	
temazepam		X	
verapamil	X		

*Inconsistent findings.
(*Source:* Adapted from Harris RZ, Benet LZ, Schwartz JB. Gender effects in Pharmacokinetics and Pharmacodynamics. *Drugs.* 1995; 50: 222–239.)

- Gender differences have been reported in the clearance of many medications, such as those listed in Table 2.2.

GENDER DIFFERENCES IN CYTOCHROME P450 SYSTEM

The cytochrome P450 system consists of hepatic enzymes that metabolize most medications and other substances.

- CYP3A4:
  - √ Predominant enzyme in cytochrome P450 system; over 60% of this system consists of CYP3A4.
  - √ Metabolizes the majority of commonly used medications (see Table 2.5).
- CYP1A1/2:
  - √ Believed to be less active in women than men.
  - √ Higher blood levels reported for women taking medications that are metabolized by CYP1A1/2, including propanolol and clozapine. In women, propanolol levels have been reported to be almost double those of men given the same dose; clozapine levels have been reported to be 35% higher than those of men given the same dose.
  - √ CYP1A1/2 activity appears to decline during pregnancy and with use of hormonal contraception.

G
E
N
D
E
R

D
I
F
F
E
D

Table 2.3. Change in Levels of Certain Medications Across the Menstrual Cycle

Medication	Change Across Menstrual Cycle
desipramine	Level rose from 73 ng/ml premenstrually to 156 ng/ml 1 week after cessation of menses
fluoxetine	No change across menstrual cycle
lithium	Inconsistent data
trazodone	Level rose from 265 ng/ml premenstrually to 551 ng/ml 1 week after cessation of menses

EFFECT OF MENSTRUAL CYCLE ON DRUG METABOLISM

- Gastrointestinal time can be slowed by as much as 30% during the high progesterone (i.e., premenstrual) phase of the menstrual cycle (see Figure 9.1).
  √ Slower gastrointestinal time can result in greater absorption of medications.
- Premenstrual edema leads to an increase in total body water with a potential decrease in blood levels of water soluble drugs (e.g., lithium), presumably through a dilutional effect.
- Effects of some psychiatric medications (Table 2.3) have been reported to vary across the menstrual cycle.
  √ Clinical significance of these data is ambiguous, because data were drawn from single subjects or small case series.

EFFECT OF PREGNANCY ON DRUG METABOLISM

The effects of pregnancy on medication concentrations are listed in Table 2.4.

- In general, the net effect of these physiological changes is a reduction in the blood levels of medications during pregnancy.

Table 2.4. Effects of Pregnancy on Medication Concentrations

Physiological Changes in Pregnancy	Effect on Medication Concentrations
Increase in hepatic metabolism	Increased medication clearance
Increase in renal clearance	Increased medication clearance
Increase in volume of distribution	Reduction in blood levels of medications
Decrease in protein binding	Increase in free fraction of protein-bound medications (e.g., valproate, carbamazepine)
Slowed gastrointestinal transit time	Increase in gastrointestinal absorption of medications.

- Medication doses may therefore need to be increased during pregnancy, particularly in the second and third trimesters.
- Pregnant women exhibit wide interindividual variation in their degree of medication clearance.
- Consider increased monitoring of medication blood levels, particularly those that must remain within a specific therapeutic window (e.g., lithium, tricyclic antidepressants, antiepileptic drugs).
- The frequency of monitoring has not been established.
  - √ Probably wise to check medication blood levels at least monthly during the second and third trimesters.
- If medication dosage is increased during pregnancy, it should probably be reduced following delivery.
  - √ This is particularly important for lithium, which can produce toxicity if blood level is even slightly above therapeutic range.
- The physiological drop in blood pressure and slowed gastrointestinal transit time in second and third trimesters exacerbate the orthostatic hypotension and constipation from tricyclic antidepressants, antipsychotic agents, and other medications.

EFFECT OF MENOPAUSAL STATUS ON DRUG METABOLISM

Drug interactions may occur between hormone replacement therapy (HRT) and other medications (see following section).

DRUG INTERACTIONS

Drug interactions may occur when two or more medications are administered concomitantly. If drug A induces the metabolism of drug B, then drug B's efficacy may be reduced. Conversely, if drug A inhibits drug B's metabolism, then drug B may produce more side effects and may reach toxic levels. Example:

- — Tamoxifen is metabolized by CYP3A4 and CYP2D6.
- — Medications that induce these enzymes (e.g., carbamazepine) should be used with caution in patients on tamoxifen.
- Table 2.5 lists substances, inhibitors, and inducers of the major cytochrome P450 enzymes involved in the metabolism of psychiatric medications.

- Drug interactions occur not only with drugs but also with certain foods (e.g., grapefruit) and nicotine.

Effect of Medications on Hormone Metabolism

- The efficacy of hormonal contraceptives and HRT can be reduced by the concomitant use of medications that induce CYP3A4 and thereby increase the metabolism of hormones.
  - √ These medications include carbamazepine, oxcarbazepine, modafinil, phenobarbital, St. John's wort, topiramate (Table 2.5).
  - √ Women should be encouraged to use a high-potency oral contraceptive (i.e., containing no less than 50 μg/day of estradiol) or an alternative method of contraception while taking these medications.
  - √ Women on HRT may need higher hormone doses to treat vasomotor symptoms.

Effect of Hormones on Medication Metabolism

- Estrogen appears to weakly inhibit 3A3/4.
- Exogenous use of estrogen (e.g., in oral contraceptives) may increase blood levels of medications that are oxidatively metabolized by 3A3/4.
- HRT does not appear to significantly alter medication levels, probably because the hormone doses are much lower than in oral contraceptives.
- Estrogen induces hepatic conjugative enzymes and may increase the metabolism of medications that are conjugated before elimination by the kidney.
- Medications that are conjugated before elimination by the kidney include:
  - √ Lamotrigine.
  - √ Lorazepam.
  - √ Oxazepam.
  - √ Temazepam.
- Through drug–drug interactions, exogenous estrogen in oral contraceptives can alter medication levels by as much as 30–60%.

Table 2.5. Substrates, Inhibitors, and Inducers of Important Cytochrome P450 Isoforms

CYP	Substrates	Inhibitors	Inducers
CYP1A2	3° amine TCAs Acetaminophen Caffeine Clozapine Haloperidol Methadone Olanzapine Phenacetin Propranolol Tacrine Theophylline Thioridazine	Cimetidine Fluoroquinolines (ciprofloxacin, norfloxacin) Fluvoxamine Mibefradil Moclobemide Grapefruit juice Ticlopidine	Carbamazepine Char-grilled meat Cigarette smoke Omeprazole Phenytoin
CYP2C9	Amitriptyline Celecoxib Fluoxetine Fluvastatin Glipizide Irbesartan Losartan NSAIDs Phenytoin Rosiglitazone S-warfarin Tolbutamide	Amiodarone Disulfiram D-propoxyphene Fluconazole Fluvastatin Fluvoxamine Miconazole Phenylbutazone Sulfaphenazole Zafirlukast	Phenytoin Rifampin Secobarbital
CYP2C19	3° amine TCAs Citalopram Diazepam Hexobarbital Indomethacin Lansoprazole Mephobarbital Moclobemlde Nelfinavir Omeprazole Phenytoin Propanolol R-warfarin Sertraline S-mephenytoin	Cimetidine Felbamate Fluoxetine Fluvoxamine Imipramine Ketoconazole Moclobemide Omeprazole Phenytoin Tranylcypromine	Rifampin
CYP2D6	2° and 3° amine TCAs Alprenolol Amphetamine Aripiprazole Beta-blockers Carvedilol Clozapine Codeine Desipramine Dextromethorphan D-fenfluramine Donepezil	Amiodarone Bupropion Celecoxib Cimetidine Fluoxetine Fluphenazine Fluvoxamine Haloperidol Hydroxybupropion Methadone Moclobemide Paroxetine	

(*Source:* Schatzberg AF, DeBattista C. Current psychotropic dosing and monitoring guidelines: 2002. *Primary Psychiatry.* 2002; 9: 34–48. Reprinted with permission.)

(*cont.*)

Table 2.5. *Continued*

CYP	Substrates	Inhibitors	Inducers
CYP2D6 (*cont*)	Fluoxetine Fluphenazine Haloperidol Hydrocodone Mexiletine Mirtazapine Nortriptyline Oxycodone Paroxetine Perphenazine Propafenone Risperidone Sertraline Tamoxifen Thioridazine Timolol Tramadol Trazodone Venlafaxine	Perphenazine Quinidine Sertraline Thioridazine	
CYP2E1	Acetaminophen Chlorzoxazone Ethanol Halothane Venlafaxine	Diethyldithiocarbamate (disulfiram metabolite)	Ethanol Isoniazid
CYP3A4	3° amine TCAs Acetaminophen Alfentanil Alprazolam Amiodarone Androgens Aripiprazole Atorvastatin Buspirone Carbamazepine Cerivastatin Citalopram Clonazepam Codeine Cyclosporine Dexamethasone Diazepam Disopyramide Donepezil Erythromycin Estrogens Ethosuximide Felodipine Fentanyl Ifosfamide Lidocaine Loratadine Lovastatin Midazolam	Amiodarone Cimetidine Clarithromycin Dexamethasone Diltiazem Erythromycin Fluconazole Fluoxetine Fluvoxamine Gestodene Grapefruit juice Indinavir Itraconazole Mibefradil Nefazodone Ritonavir Saquinavir Sertraline Troleandomycin Verapamil	Barbiturates Carbamazepine Dexamethasone Felbamate Ketoconazole Modafinil Oxcarbazepine Phenobarbital Phenytoin Pioglitazone Primidone Rifampin St. John's wort Topiramate

(cont.)

Table 2.5. *Continued*

CYP	Substrates	Inhibitors	Inducers
CYP3A4 (cont)	Mirtazapine Nefazodone Nifedipine Nimodipine Nisoldipine Nitrendipine Norethindrone Omeprazole Progesterone Propafenone Protease inhibitors Quetiapine Quinidine Sertraline Sibutramine Sildenafil Simvastatin Sufentanil Tacrolimus Tamoxifen Testosterone Tiagabine Trazodone Triazolam Verapamil Vinblastine Vincristine Ziprasidone Zolpidem		

(*Source:* Adapted from Schatzberg AF, DeBattista C. Current psychotropic dosing and monitoring guidelines. *Primary Psychiatry.* 2002;47: 34–48.)

GENDER DIFFERENCES

3. Depressive Disorders

INTRODUCTION

Epidemiological studies consistently report a higher prevalence of depression in women than men. The relatively high rate of depression during women's reproductive years accounts for this gender difference; among prepubertal girls and postmenopausal (including elderly) women, rates of depression are not higher than their male counterparts. A number of explanations has been suggested for the elevated risk of depression among reproductive-aged women, including psychosocial explanations such as exposure to trauma and chronic stressors, cognitive styles such as a tendency toward ruminative thinking, and biological explanations such as the impact of reproductive hormones on the synthesis and inactivation of neurotransmitters.

The clinical manifestation and course of depression also vary somewhat by gender. Depressed women are more likely to report anxiety, guilt, and indecisiveness, whereas depressed men express more self-criticism. Depressed men tend to experience insomnia and diminished appetite ("classic" neurovegetative symptoms), while depressed women are more likely to present with "atypical," or reverse, neurovegetative symptoms (i.e., increased sleep and appetite). In addition, women are more likely to experience a seasonal pattern, typically with heightened vulnerability to depression during winter months.

Few studies have examined gender and age differences in response to antidepressant medications. The largest study on this question reported that premenopausal women were more likely to respond to sertraline than imipramine, whereas men responded better to imipramine. Postmenopausal women showed similar rates of response to both medications. Two additional studies have reported a better response to fluoxetine among premenopausal women compared to postmenopausal women. Researchers have speculated that women's estrogen status may influence their treatment response to antidepressants. However, two recent reports that analyzed data from a total of 17 clinical trials found that gender and age did not appear to influence response to antidepressants. Hopefully, future studies will help shed light on the impact of gender and age—and menopausal status—on response to antidepressants.

General considerations in treating depression in women include obtaining thyroid testing, particularly in patients who report symptoms suggestive of hypothyroidism (see p. 6). Thyroid disorders occur more frequently in women than men and may contribute to mood instability. Women > 40 years of age are particularly at risk for thyroid dysfunction. It is also important to evaluate whether mood symptoms vary in a seasonal pattern.

Depression can occur in either an episodic or chronic course. Some studies report that women are more likely than men to experience recurrences and to develop a chronic form of the illness. For the episodic form of depression, the principal predictor of further recurrence is the number of prior episodes. The greater the number of prior episodes, the greater the likelihood of a future episode. Additional risk factors for recurrent depression include long duration of depressive episodes, history of premenstrual dysphoric disorder (PMDD), family history of depression, comorbid anxiety disorder or substance abuse, and onset of depression after age 60.

Patients also differ in the extent to which the depressive episodes are precipitated by life stresses—for example, relationship difficulties, financial problems, death or severe illness of a loved one—versus emerging spontaneously without an obvious precipitating stressor. Women are more likely to become depressed in the face of marital conflict, child-care difficulties, and other forms of family distress, whereas men are generally more vulnerable to employment-related stress. Stress-precipitated depressive episodes seem to respond as well to antidepressants as do episodes that arise spontaneously. The presence of significant life stressors, however, should encourage the consideration of psychotherapy in addition to the antidepressant treatment.

Thoughts of suicide can occur among severely depressed individuals. It is incumbent on clinicians to evaluate suicidal potential in all patients with significant depressive symptoms. Most serious suicide attempts among women involve medication overdoses. Therefore, clinicians should be alert to the amount and potential lethality of medications available to the patient at home.

Comorbid psychiatric disorders can complicate the evaluation and treatment of depression. Women are more likely to experience comorbid anxiety and eating disorders, whereas men are more likely to suffer from comorbid alcohol and substance abuse. Comorbid psychiatric disorders usually predict worse treatment outcomes.

The incidence of depression (both major and minor) in pregnant women is approximately 10%, comparable to that in nonpregnant women. Risk factors for depression in pregnancy include conflict with the baby's father, lack of social support, previous history of depression, and low socioeconomic status. Potential risks of untreated depression in pregnant women include poor nutrition; inadequate weight gain (a strong predictor of infant birth weight); use of alcohol, nicotine, and illicit substances; and, in severe cases, suicidality. Depressed women who are pregnant or attempting to conceive should be encouraged to initiate psychotherapy if they are not already obtaining it. One form of therapy that has been particularly well-studied in pregnant women is interpersonal psychotherapy, which focuses on the impact of role transitions and interpersonal interactions.

Postpartum depression refers to a major depressive episode following childbirth. DSM-IV defines "postpartum-onset" as occurring within 4 weeks of delivery. However, most studies of postpartum depression included women whose depression occurred within 1–6 months following delivery. Women with previous histories of major depression represent the group at greatest risk for postpartum depression. Additional risk factors include marital conflict, stressful life events, social disadvantage, and child-care stresses (e.g., colicky infant; infant with multiple health problems; presence of other young children in the home). Postpartum depression is a condition that affects approximately 12% of new mothers. Given that 4–5 million women give birth in the United States each year, this rate translates to hundreds of thousands of women. Postpartum depression is frequently complicated by comorbid anxiety and obsessional symptoms (e.g., about the infant's safety). Most cases of postpartum depression respond well to treatment, which may include psychotherapy, group support, antidepressant medications, and, if necessary, medications to treat anxiety and insomnia. Bright light therapy also may be helpful.

Postpartum depression should be distinguished from the postpartum "blues," a mild mood syndrome that many new mothers experience following delivery. Symptoms include moodiness, crying spells, and generalized anxiety. Postpartum blues typically remit over the course of 1–2 weeks. Postpartum depression also should be distinguished from postpartum *psychosis*, a rare but serious condition affecting approximately 0.1–0.2% of new mothers (see Chapter 4). Women with histories of bipolar or schizoaffective disorder are at greatest risk.

Effective treatment of postpartum depression benefits not only the mother but also the child. Depressed mothers are more likely to be withdrawn and irritable and to exhibit negative parenting behaviors, such as yelling and shaking the child. Several studies have demonstrated that maternal depression in the first year after delivery is associated with a negative and potentially sustained impact on children's cognitive and emotional development. Children of depressed mothers tend to have more difficulty with emotional regulation, develop lower self-esteem, and show more aggressive behavior toward their parents and peers. Boys are more vulnerable than girls to the adverse developmental impact of maternal depression. Children are at greatest risk if their mothers are of low socioeconomic status and have low levels of education. Children of mothers who experienced depression in the child's first year of life appear to be at greater risk for adverse cognitive outcomes, compared to children who were older when their mothers experienced depression. Multiple relapses of maternal depression also increase the risk for poor cognitive outcomes in the children. Underscoring the importance of intervention, preliminary research has found that treatment of maternal depression leads to improvements in children's developmental outcomes. Early interventions are essential, because the degree of risk to children appears to be related to the duration of the mother's depression. Prompt treatment of maternal depression significantly reduces the likelihood of adverse consequences to the child.

Perimenopause describes the transitional time between a woman's reproductive years and menopause. Most women do not experience an increase in depressive symptoms during the perimenopausal transition. However, certain factors place women at risk for depression during this period, including (1) a history of depression, (2) a history of premenstrual dysphoric disorder, (3) severe vasomotor symptoms, and (4) psychosocial stressors (e.g., marital conflict, burdensome caregiving responsibilities). Negative expectations of menopause also increase the likelihood that a woman will experience a low mood through the perimenopausal transition.

Depression in elderly women is frequently overlooked, because clinicians tend to focus on patients' medical problems and physical disabilities. Screening and treatment of depression in this population is of great importance, as depression in elderly women significantly raises their risk for disabilities in mobility and activities of daily living. These disabilities, in turn, exacerbate depression and social isolation, producing a downward spiral of frailty and failure to thrive. Depressive symptoms are more common in the "old-old" than in younger elderly patients (> 20% vs. < 10%). This greater prevalence rate appears to result from the higher proportion of women in this population, their greater likelihood of physical and cognitive impairments, and their generally lower socioeconomic status.

ANTIDEPRESSANTS

- 26 antidepressants are available in the United States.
- The four major classes of antidepressants are:
  √ Selective serotonin reuptake inhibitors (SSRIs);
  √ Serotonin–norepinephrine reuptake inhibitors (SNRIs);
  √ Tricyclic antidepressants (TCAs);
  √ Monoamine oxidase inhibitors (MAOIs).
- Four other medications are classified as novel agents:
  √ Bupropion.
  √ Mirtazapine.
  √ Nefazodone.
  √ Trazodone.
    □ These are biologically different from each other (with the exception of trazodone and nefazodone, which are relatively similar) and from the four major classes of antidepressants.

Choosing an Antidepressant

- Side-effect profile:
  √ May be used therapeutically (e.g., prescribe a sedating antidepressant for an anxious/agitated patient or prescribe an activating medication for a psychomotor-retarded patient).

□ Helps to prevent medication nonadherence and alleviate some symptoms but does not predict response to the antidepressant.

- Ease of administration (e.g., daily dosing vs. bid or tid)
- Patient's and family's history of past response
- Medical considerations.
- Safety in overdose:
  √ Patients who express suicidal thoughts should not be given medications that are potentially fatal in overdose without ensuring that another person keeps the medications safe and dispenses them in small amounts.
- Cost:
  √ Depends on patient's financial means, insurance coverage, potential formulary issues (via insurance).
    □ Fluoxetine, fluvoxamine, bupropion-IR, mirtazapine, trazodone, and most TCAs are available in generic form; other antidepressants will also be available generically over the next few years.
- For women of reproductive age:
  √ If patient plans to conceive in near future, try to use medication with safety data in pregnancy.
- Pre- vs. postmenopausal status:
  √ Some studies report that premenopausal women, but not postmenopausal women, respond better to serotonergic antidepressants.
- Comorbid psychiatric conditions:
  √ For example, if the patient suffers from comorbid PMDD (Chapter 7) or an eating disorder (Chapter 8), serotonergic antidepressants may be preferable.
- Potential for drug interactions (Chapter 2)
- Neurotransmitter specificity (e.g., serotonergic agents to treat obsessional symptoms or poor impulse control; noradrenergic agents to improve concentration and attention).
- Blood level considerations (e.g., with TCAs, blood levels can help guide dosing and ensure compliance).

Selective Serotonin Reuptake Inhibitors (SSRIs)

- Six agents are available:
  √ citalopram (Celexa).
  √ S-citalopram (Lexapro).
  √ fluoxetine (Prozac).
  √ fluvoxamine (Luvox).

✓ paroxetine (Paxil).

✓ sertraline (Zoloft).

- Agents are more alike than different in their efficacy and side-effect profiles.
- Presumed dominant biological effect for all agents is increase in serotonin function in central nervous system.
- S-citalopram, released in 2002, is a stereoisomer of citalopram.
  ✓ Similar to parent compound but prescribed at lower dose.

Dosing

- Consider starting at half dose for first 3–7 days to decrease side effects (see Table 3.2).
- Suggested starting and target doses are shown in Table 3.1.

Table 3.1. Antidepressants Available in the United States

Generic Name (Trade Name)	Typical Starting Dose (mg)	Usual Dosage Range (mg/day)
Selective Serotonin Reuptake Inhibitors		
citalopram (Celexa)	10–20	20–60
S-citalopram (Lexapro)	5–10	10–30
fluoxetine (Prozac)	10–20	10–80
fluvoxamine (Luvox)	25–50	100–300
paroxetine (Paxil)	10–20	20–60
sertraline (Zoloft)	25–50	50–200
Serotonin Norepinephrine Reuptake Inhibitors		
venlafaxine (Effexor)	37.5–75	150–300
duloxetine (Cymbalta)	20–60	40–120
Tricyclics and Related Compounds		
amitriptyline (Elavil, Endep)	25–50	100–300
amoxapine (Asendin)	50–100	150–400
clomipramine (Anafranil)	25–50	100–250
desipramine (Norpramin, Pertofrane)	25–50	100–300
doxepin (Sinequan, Adapin)	25–50	100–300
imipramine (Tofranil)	25–50	100–300
maprotiline (Ludiomil)	25–50	100–225
nortriptyline (Aventyl, Pamelor)	10–25	50–150
protriptyline (Vivactil)	10	15–60
trimipramine (Surmontil)	25–50	100–300
Monoamine Oxidase Inhibitors (MAOIs)		
isocarboxazid (Marplan)	10–20	30–60
phenelzine (Nardil)	15–30	30–90
selegiline (Eldepryl)	10	20–60
tranylcypromine (Parnate)	10–20	30–60
Other Antidepressants		
bupropion (Wellbutrin)	100–150	300–450
mirtazapine (Remeron)	15–30	15–60
nefazodone (Serzone)	50	400–600
trazodone (Desyrel)	50	150–400

DEPRESSIVE DISORDERS

Serotonin Norepinephrine Reuptake Inhibitors (SNRIs)

- Two agents available:
  - √ venlafaxine (Effexor).
  - √ duloxetine (Cymbalta).
- Inhibit the reuptake of serotonin and norepinephrine.

Venlafaxine (Effexor)

- At low doses (< 150 mg/day), predominant effect is strong selective increase in serotonin function, identical to SSRIs.
- At higher dose, gradual increase in noradrenergic (norepinephrine) effect while preserving serotonergic effect, thereby becoming a dual-action antidepressant.
- Available as IR (immediate release) and XR (extended release) forms.
- No important pharmacokinetic interactions.
- Very short half-life; therefore, high risk of withdrawal symptoms (see Table 3.8).
  - √ If discontinuing, taper very slowly (e.g., over 2–4 weeks).

Dosing
- Begin at 37.5 mg capsules, one to two tablets/capsules daily; increase to 150 mg/day and then wait 3 weeks.
- XR prescribed once daily; IR usually prescribed twice daily.

Potential Side Effects
- Same as SSRIs (see Table 3.2).
- IR form associated with far more nausea than XR form.
- Increase in blood pressure
  - √ Dose related, starting at dose of 150 mg/day.
    - □ Affects approximately 9% of patients treated with high dose (> 300 mg/day).
    - □ Pretreatment hypertension (if treated) *not* a contraindication.

Duloxetine (Cymbalta)

- Reuptake inhibitor of norepinephrine and serotonin, at starting and usual doses.
- Scheduled for release in 2004.
- Demonstrated efficacy for depression.
- Half-time = 12 hours.
  - √ Nonetheless, effective in once daily dosing.

Table 3.2. Common SSRI Side Effects

Side Effect	Relative Incidence Across SSRIs
Nausea	Slightly more common with fluvoxamine
Stimulation	Fluoxetine > sertraline > S-citalopram > citalopram > paroxetine > fluvoxamine
Sedation	Fluvoxamine > paroxetine > citalopram, S-citalopram > sertraline > fluoxetine
Sexual side effects • Include delayed time to orgasm, anorgasmia, decreased libido • Generally do not remit over time	Similar prevalence across agents
Apathy	Similar prevalence across agents
Weight gain • Late onset, typically 3–12 months after treatment has begun • Ranges from 5–30 lbs	May be somewhat greater with paroxetine
Cognitive dysfunction • Short-term memory deficits, word-finding difficulties	Similar prevalence across agents.
Elimination half-life (see Table 3.8) correlates with likelihood of withdrawal symptoms after antidepressant discontinuation	5-week washout for fluoxetine, 10–14 day washout for all other SSRIs
Withdrawal symptoms include dizziness, paresthesias, dysesthesias, irritability, insomnia	Least with fluoxetine (longest half-life), most with paroxetine (shortest half-life)
Hyperprolactinemia • May produce breast enlargement, galactorrhea (milky nipple discharge) • May produce irregular menses or amenorrhea	Not well-studied Theoretically, can occur with any SSRI Risk may be lower with sertraline because its dopaminergic effects may offset the serotonergic elevation of prolactin
Excess perspiration	Probably similar prevalence across agents
P450 effects	Fluoxetine and paroxetine strongly inhibit P450 2D6 enzymes and can therefore increase blood levels of concomitantly prescribed tricyclic antidepressants. They also inhibit 3A4 to a lesser degree. Sertraline inhibits 2D6, but to a lesser degree than fluoxetine and paroxetine. Citalopram and S-citalopram have few pharmacokinetic interactions

DEPRESSIVE DISORDERS

Table 3.3. Treatment of Antidepressant Side Effects

Side Effect	Treatment
Nausea	• Take dose after meals • Wait for accommodation (nausea often remits quickly)
Stimulation	• Take dose in morning • Wait for accommodation to occur (common over days to weeks) • Switch to less activating agent • Add trazodone or benzodiazepines for insomnia • Add benzodiazepines or gabapentin for daytime anxiety
Sedation (sedation can be used for daytime tranquilizer effect; if so, prescribe in divided daily doses)	• Take dose in evening • Wait for accomodation to occur • Switch to more activating agent • Add a stimulating medication (e.g., modafanil)

Sexual side effects	• Add buspirone (Buspar) 20–80 mg/day—can be used as needed
	• Add sildenafil (Viagra) 50–100 mg/day—can be used as needed
	  √ More effective for arousal and orgasm dysfunction than for libido
	• Add bupropion (Wellbutrin)
	  √ May require 300 mg/day
	  √ Usually prescribed daily
	• Add stimulants (e.g., methylphenidate, d-amphetamine typically prescribed on as-needed basis
	• Discontinue medication on weekends ("weekend holiday")

Apathy	• Reduce dose • Switch to another agent • Add a stimulant (e.g., modafanil, methylphenidate, d-amphetamine)
Weight gain	• Add a stimulant (e.g., modafanil, methylphenidate, d-amphetamine) • Add topiramate 50–200 mg/day
Cognitive dysfunction	• Reduce dose • Switch to another agent • Add a stimulant (e.g., modafanil, methylphenidate, d-amphetamine)
Withdrawal symptoms	• Slow taper (i.e., over 2–4 weeks) • If needed, switch to fluoxetine (longest half-life SSRI) for 3 days and then taper
Hyperprolactinemia	• Reduce dose • Switch to another agent • Administer low doses of dopamine agonists (see Chapter 6)
Excess perspiration	• Reduce dose • Add benztropine 0.5–2 mg/day

(cont.)

Table 3.3. *Continued*

Side Effect	Treatment
P450 effects	• Adjust medication dosage depending on whether interactions with other agents inhibit or induce its metabolism • Switch to another agent
New-onset hypertension (e.g., with venlafaxine)	• Switch agents • Add antihypertensive agent.
Seizures (e.g., with bupropion, clomipramine)	• Prescribe in divided doses (especially bupropion) • Prescribe sustained-release formulation (for bupropion) • Do not exceed recommended dose • Do not prescribe to patients at risk of seizures (e.g., active eating disorders; history of head trauma; history of epilepsy)

Dosing
• See Table 3.1.

Potential Side effects
• Most common:
  √ Nausea-Accommodation to the nausea occurs quickly in many patients.
  √ Dizziness.
  √ Dry mouth.
  √ Fatigue.
  √ Constipation.
• Rate of discontinuation due to side effects similar to SSRIs.
• Pre-release studies indicate no propensity for hypertension.

Tricyclic Antidepressants (TCAs)

• Ten agents available:
  √ amitriptyline (Elavil, Endep).
  √ amoxapine (Asendin).
  √ clomipramine (Anafranil).
  √ desipramine (Norpramin, Pertofrane).
  √ doxepin (Sinequan, Adapin).
  √ imipramine (Tofranil).
  √ maprotiline (Ludiomil).
  √ nortriptyline (Aventyl, Pamelor).
  √ protriptyline (Vivactil).
  √ trimipramine (Surmontil).

- Oldest class of antidepressants.
- Seldom used now because of safety concerns and tolerability issues, although as effective as newer agents.
- Biological effects: reuptake inhibition of serotonin, norepinephrine, or both.
- Serotonergic effects are generally weak compared to SSRIs or venlafaxine, except for clomipramine which is highly serotonergic.

Dosing
See Table 3.1 (p. 37).

Potential Side Effects
- Anticholinergic effects (less likely with nortriptyline, desipramine, maprotiline) include:
  √ Dry mouth.
  √ Blurry vision.
  √ Urinary retention.
  √ Constipation.
- Sedation.
- Stimulation: mostly with noradrenergic tricyclics (imipramine, desipramine).
- Orthostatic hypotension: less likely with nortriptyline, desipramine, maprotiline.
- Weight gain.
- Alterations in cardiac conduction
  √ Can be potentially dangerous in patients with heart disease.
  √ Very dangerous/easily fatal in overdose.
- Side effects differ across tricyclic agents (see Table 3.6).

Serum Levels
- For the following tricylic antidepressants, plasma levels correlate with efficacy.
- Therapeutic ranges:
  √ Desipramine: > 125 ng/ml.
  √ Imipramine: 200–350 ng/ml.
  √ Nortriptyline: 50–150 ng/ml.
  √ Amitriptyline: 95–140 ng/ml.
- Obtain levels 10–14 hours after last dose, once the patient has been at a steady dose for at least 1 week.
- Estrogen-containing hormonal contraceptives can increase blood levels of tricyclic antidepressants (through inhibiting CYP3A4—see Chapter 2).

Monoamine Oxidase Inhibitors (MAOIs)

- Four agents available:
  - √ isocarboxazid (Marplan).
  - √ phenelzine (Nardil).
  - √ selegiline (Eldepryl).
  - √ tranylcypromine (Parnate).
- Mechanism of action:
  - √ All agents inhibit the intracellular enzyme monoamine oxidase (MAO), which deaminates a number of neurotransmitters, including dopamine, norepinephrine, and serotonin.
  - √ By inhibiting deamination, these medications enhance the function of these neurotransmitter systems.
- All currently available MAOIs in the United States are irreversible in their binding to MAO.
- Reversible MAO inhibitors (RIMAs) are available in Europe.
  - √ These have fewer side effects and no dietary restrictions (see Table 3.4).
- Effective in all types of depressions; especially effective for atypical depression.
- Used infrequently because of side effects and dietary restrictions.

Dosing

- The dose may be consolidated, if tolerated.
- Progress from starting dose (see Table 3.1) to full dose over 1–2 weeks.

Table 3.4. Dietary Restrictions for Patients on Monoamine Oxidase Inhibitors

Food and Beverages to Avoid Completely	Foods or Beverages to be Used in Moderation
Cheese—all kinds except cottage cheese, ricotta, and cream cheese	Canned or packeted soups
Smoked or pickled fish (*canned tuna okay*)	
Fermented meats, such as summer sausage, salami, mortadella	Other alcoholic beverages
Sauerkraut	Yogurt
Yeast/protein extracts, such as Marmite and Bovril spreads	Sour cream
Red wines, especially chianti	Avocados
Imported or tap beers	Raspberries
Sherry, vermouth	
White wine and champagne okay	
Fava or broad bean pods (Italian green beans); *the beans themselves okay*	
Beef or chicken liver (unless absolutely fresh)	
Overripe figs or overripe bananas (*young bananas with white pulp okay*)	
Soy products	

Potential Side Effects
- Orthostatic hypotension.
- Insomnia.
- Daytime fatigue/energy slumps.
- Sexual dysfunction.
- Weight gain with isocarboxazid, phenelzine.

Mandatory Dietary Restrictions
- Certain foods and medications ingested by patients on MAOIs will cause severe, potentially life threatening reactions.
- These foods and medications are absolutely contraindicated for patients on MAOIs and for 2 weeks after stopping the MAOI.
  - √ Except for venlafaxine and nefazodone, for which the washout is 1 week, and fluoxetine, which requires a 5-week washout.
- Two types of reactions may occur:
  - √ Hypertensive crises
    - □ Caused by foods containing tyramine or other pressor amines, and medications with sympathomimetic properties.
    - □ Thought to occur because the enzyme MAO in gut, liver, and brain deaminates tyramine and other pressor amines found in foods.
    - □ With MAO inhibition, these amines increase blood pressure.
  - √ Serotonin syndrome
    - □ Caused by medication combinations with strong serotonergic properties.
    - □ Since MAOIs also strongly enhance serotonergic function, excessive serotonergic activity in the hypothalamus ensues, resulting in serotonin syndrome, characterized by fever, muscle rigidity, hypotension, high fever, and mental status changes.
- All patients on MAOIs must be given a written list of contraindicated foods and medications.
- Table 3.4 lists the dietary restrictions; Table 3.5 lists the contraindicated medications.
- All antibiotics are safe, as are aspirin, plain Tylenol, Advil, and Motrin.
- Patients should check with their psychiatrists before taking any other medicines.
- Patients must also tell their doctors or dentists that they are taking an MAOI.

Table 3.5. Medications to Avoid With Monoamine Oxidase Inhibitors

Medications with Stimulant Properties Causing Hypertensive Reactions:

- Virtually all cold, cough, or sinus medications (except pure antihistamines such as Benadryl, Chlortrimeton, or Allegra)
- Weight-reducing or pep pills
- Asthma inhalants (except for steroid sprays or Intal)
- Epinephrine in local anesthesia, such as is used in dental work (local anesthesia itself is safe)
- Cocaine
- Amphetamines, speed
- Other antidepressants (except in special circumstances)

Medications Causing Serotonin (Hyperpyrexic) Syndrome:

- Antidepressants with strong serotonergic effects, including:
  - √ clomipramine (Anafranil)
  - √ citalopram (Celexa, Lexapro)
  - √ duloxetine (Cymbalta)
  - √ fluoxetine (Prozac)
  - √ fluvoxamine (Luvox)
  - √ nefazodone (Serzone)
  - √ paroxetine (Paxil)
  - √ sertraline (Zoloft)
  - √ venlafaxine (Effexor)
- Some opiates:
  - √ meperidine (Demerol)
  - √ dextromethorphan (found in many cold and cough preparations, usually labeled as DM)

- Table 3.6 compares the relative likelihood of side effects across antidepressants.

Other Antidepressants

Bupropion (Wellbutrin)

- Predominantly dopaminergic and noradrenergic effects.
- Available as immediate, sustained, and extended-release forms (IR, SR, XL).

Dosing
- With IR form:
  - √ Start with 100 mg bid, increasing to 300 mg/day.
  - √ Prescribe maximum of 150 mg/dose, with maximum daily dose of 450 mg, thereby requiring tid dosing.
- With SR form:
  - √ Start with either 100 mg bid or 150 mg once daily, increasing to 300 mg/day.
  - √ Prescribe maximum of 200 mg/dose, with maximum daily dose of 400 mg, thereby requiring tid dosing.
- With XL form:
  - √ Start with 150 mg once daily, increasing to 450 mg once daily.

Table 3.6. Relative Likelihood of Specific Side Effects Across Antidepressants

Name (trade name)	Stimulation	Sedation	Postural Hypotension	Anticholinergic Effects
Selective Serotonin Reuptake Inhibitors				
citalopram (Celexa)	+	+	0	0
S-citalopram (Lexapro)	+-++	+	0	0
fluoxetine (Prozac)	+++	0-+	0	0
fluvoxamine (Luvox)	+	++	0	0
paroxetine (Paxil)	+	++	0	+
sertraline (Zoloft)	++	0-+	0	0
Novel Antidepressants				
bupropion (Wellbutrin)	++	0	0	0
mirtazapine (Remeron)	0	+++	0	0
nefazodone (Serzone)	0	+++	++	0
trazodone (Desyrel)	0	+++	+++	0
venlafaxine (Effexor)	+	+	0	0
Tricyclics and Related Compounds				
amitriptyline (Elavil, Endep)	0	+++	+++	+++
amoxapine (Asendin)	0	+	++	+
clomipramine (Anafranil)	0	+++	+++	+++
desipramine (Norpramin, Pertofrane)	+	+	+	+
doxepin (Sinequan, Adapin)	0	+++	+++	++
imipramine (Tofranil)	+	++	+++	++
maprotiline (Ludiomil)	+	++	+	+
nortriptyline (Aventyl, Pamelor)	0	++	+	+
protriptyline (Vivactil)	+	+	+++	+++
trimipramine (Surmontil)	0	+++	++	+++
Monoamine Oxidase Inhibitors (MAOIs)				
isocarboxazid (Marplan)	+	++	+++	+
phenelzine (Nardil)	+	++	+++	+
selegiline (Eldepryl)	+	+	++	+
tranylcypromine (Parnate)	++	+	+++	+

0 none; 0-+ minimal; + mild; ++ moderate; +++ significant.

Potential Side Effects

- All related to stimulation effects:
  - √ Anxiety.
  - √ Insomnia.
  - √ Tremulousness.
  - √ Headache.
- Seizures:
  - √ Rare.
  - √ Bupropion produces a slightly greater risk of seizures than other antidepressants.
  - √ Contraindicated in those with lowered seizure thresholds, such as patients with active eating disorders or with history of seizure disorder.

✓ SR form is associated with a lower seizure risk than IR form in daily doses up to 300 mg.
- No weight gain.
- No sexual side effects.
- Virtually never sedating.

Mirtazapine (Remeron)
- Biological effects are complex: Most important is thought to be presynaptic alpha-2 blocking (which therefore enhances adrenergic function), with secondary enhancement of serotonin activity.
- Increasingly used in geriatric depression.
- Used primarily for anxious, agitated, insomnic, or anorexic depressions.
- Available in Soltab form (orally dissolvable).

Dosing
- Start at dose of 15, 30, or 45 mg/day, typically prescribed in evening.
- Although *PDR* maximum dose is 45 mg/day, studies and clinical experience have safely used doses up to 90 mg/day.

Potential Side Effects
- Sedation.
- Weight gain.

Nefazodone (Serzone)
- Most prominent biological effect is postsynaptic serotonin-2 blockade.
- Weak noradrenergic effects and weak serotonin reuptake inhibition.

Dosing
- Start at low dose (25–50 mg/day) and gradually increase as tolerated.
- Low doses (i.e., 50–300 mg/day) are primarily anxiolytic.
- Full antidepressant dose: 400–600 mg/day.
- Blood levels of nefazodone are reportedly higher in elderly women than young women or men of any age, so elderly women should probably receive lower doses to avoid excessive side effects.

Potential Side Effects
- Sedation.
- Nausea.

- Dizziness.
- Dry mouth.
- Hepatotoxicity.
  - √ Rare.
  - √ Seen idiosyncratically, mostly in the first 6 months of treatment.
  - √ Rare; estimated prevalence 1/250,000 patients/year.
  - √ No reliable warnings occur prior to clinical symptoms.
  - √ Stop medication immediately if signs of hepatitis.
- No sexual side effects.
- No weight gain.

Trazodone (Desyrel)
- Rarely used as antidepressant; prescribed primarily as a hypnotic.

PHASES OF TREATMENT

Acute

- For the vast majority of depressions, all antidepressants are equivalently effective.
- Potential exceptions are:
  - √ Very severe depressions (typically those hospitalized or being considered for electroconvulsive therapy [ECT]) may respond less well to SSRIs than to other classes.
  - √ Atypical depressions may respond better to MAO inhibitors and possibly to SSRIs.
  - √ Some studies have reported that women of reproductive age respond better to SSRIs than TCAs.
- Response is typically defined as > 50% improvement in symptoms, measured in research studies using the Hamilton Rating Scale for Depression (HRSD).
  - √ Response rate is 60% for patients who complete a full trial of antidepressants (i.e., minimum 4–6 weeks of treatment).
  - √ Dropout rate is 10–15% with newer agents; 15–25% with older agents.
- Remission is defined as virtually complete response (HRSD score < 8).
  - √ Remission rate is 35–45% for patients who complete a full trial of antidepressants.
- Efficacy typically occurs within 2–6 weeks of initiating treatment.

- A subset of patients responds more quickly (within the first week) with decreased anxiety, improved sleep, decreased irritability (possibly more common with SSRIs).

Continuation

- Prevents relapse into same episode for which treatment was instituted.
- Once treatment is effective (i.e., 80% or more improvement in depressive symptoms), keep patients on antidepressant for 6–9 months at the acute treatment dose.
- If maintenance treatment is not appropriate (e.g., after first acute episode), taper antidepressant over 1 month (or more slowly) to avoid both sudden relapse and/or withdrawal symptoms.
- For dysthymic disorder, 1–2 year continuation treatment and then consider possible antidepressant withdrawal.

Maintenance

- Prevents recurrent episodes of depression.
- Consider the following factors in deciding on maintenance treatment:
  √ Number of depressive episodes.
    □ Consider maintenance treatment after three or more recurrences.
  √ Frequency of depressive episodes.
  √ Severity of depressive episodes.
  √ Response of prior episodes to treatment.
  √ Depressive recurrence after antidepressant withdrawal in the past.
- For maintenance treatment, use same dose as for acute treatment.
  √ Exception is when side effects are intolerable; then decrease dose as little as necessary.

TREATMENT CONSIDERATIONS FOR WOMEN OF REPRODUCTIVE AGE

- Obtain initial menstrual history:
  √ Typical cycle length.
  √ Typical duration of menses.

- Monitor patient's symptoms in relation to her menstrual cycle.
  - ✓ If patient experiences recurrent premenstrual relapse or exacerbation of depression, consider increasing medication dose by 50% at midcycle.
  - ✓ Blood levels of antidepressants have been reported to vary across the menstrual cycle.
    - □ If the patient reports a recurrent relapse or exacerbation of depression, consider measuring the antidepressant concentration premenstrually and in the follicular phase of the menstrual cycle (for medications with well-established therapeutic ranges, such as TCAs).
    - □ If the serum antidepressant concentration is found to drop premenstrually, consider increasing the antidepressant dosage at midcycle.
- Monitor whether patient's menstrual cycle changes following initiation of antidepressant.
  - ✓ Consider instructing patients to chart menstrual cycles (e.g., with chart such as Figure 7.1,) after initiating certain medications.
  - ✓ Serotonergic antidepressants can increase prolactin levels and produce irregular menses and amenorrhea (with the possible exception of sertraline, because its dopaminergic effects may offset the impact on prolactin).
- For heterosexual women who take antidepressants and are sexually active:
  - ✓ Obtain immediate pregnancy test if recent unprotected sex.
  - ✓ OTC pregnancy test 99% accurate at 12–14 days postconception.
  - ✓ Educate about risks of medication exposure to fetus if patient becomes pregnant.
  - ✓ Encourage patients to use contraception regularly if they do not wish to conceive.

TREATMENT OF DEPRESSION DURING PREGNANCY

- Whenever possible, review treatment options during pregnancy prior to a woman's discontinuation of contraception.
- If a patient is likely to remain psychiatrically stable, even without medications, for several weeks or longer, consider tapering and discontinuing the medication before she attempts to conceive.

- Certain medications should be tapered rather than stopped abruptly to avoid withdrawal symptoms (e.g., paroxetine, venlafaxine).
- If a woman has a history of severe relapse of depression following medication discontinuation, the antidepressant may need to be continued throughout the pregnancy.
- In general, patients with a previous episode of depression face approximately a 25–30% risk of relapse of depression over the next year.
- Additional risk factors to consider are presence of psychosocial stressors that increase the likelihood of relapse (e.g., financial hardship, work-related stresses, marital conflict—including domestic violence, the incidence of which escalates during pregnancy).
- Review measures that may reduce likelihood of relapse (e.g., psychotherapy; couples counseling; change in work schedule; assistance with child-care responsibilities).
- When medications are used in pregnancy: Maintain the lowest dosage and fewest medications necessary for control of symptoms.
- Whenever possible, try to postpone use of medications until after 12th gestational week; this is particularly important for medications with limited safety data in pregnancy.
- Gestational age is dated from the time of a woman's last menstrual period, *not* from the date of conception.
  - √ Conception typically occurs approximately 2 weeks after a menstrual period.
  - √ Therefore, the actual fetal age is about 2 weeks less than the gestational age.
  - √ The 12th gestational week corresponds to a fetal age of approximately 10 weeks.
- Medication doses may require adjustment during pregnancy because of increased liver metabolism, decreased protein binding, and greater volume of distribution (see Chapter 2).
- No antidepressant currently has FDA approval for use during pregnancy.
- FDA use-in-pregnancy categories for medications are listed in Table 1.4.
- FDA use-in-pregnancy ratings for antidepressants are listed in Table 3.7 use in pregnancy ratings for additional medications are listed in Table 1.5.

DEPRESSIVE DISORDERS

Table 3.7. FDA Use-in-Pregnancy Ratings for Antidepressants

Medication	Rating
amitriptyline (Elavil, Endep)	D
bupropion (Wellbutrin)	B
citalopram (Celexa, Lexapro)	C
clomipramine (Anafranil)	C
desipramine (Norpramin, Pertofrane)	C
doxepin (Adapin, Sinequan)	C
fluoxetine (Prozac, Sarafem)	C
fluvoxamine (Luvox)	C
imipramine (Tofranil)	D
mirtazapine (Remeron)	C
nefazodone (Serzone)	C
nortriptyline (Aventyl, Pamelor)	D
paroxetine (Paxil)	C
sertraline (Zoloft)	C
trazodone (Desyrel)	C
venlafaxine (Effexor)	C

✓ Medications carrying an FDA Pregnancy Category B rating are not necessarily safer to use in pregnancy than medications with Pregnancy Category C labeling.

✓ Medications for which no human data exist may receive the Category B rating if animal studies have not found a fetal risk.

✓ Category C-labeled medications, for which human data show low risk, may be preferable to Category B-labeled medications, for which there are no human data.

- The decision to use an antidepressant during pregnancy ultimately depends on:
  ✓ The risks of continued depression on the mother and fetus.
  ✓ Research findings on the safety/risks of medication use in pregnancy.

- Research data primarily come from:
  ✓ Naturalistic studies.
  ✓ Reports of pregnancy outcomes from callers to Teratogen Information Services (TIS).
  ✓ Single case reports or small case series.
  ✓ Pharmaceutical company pregnancy registries.

- Research data often involve trade name products (e.g., Prozac [fluoxetine]). Because generic formulations may be slightly different, it is best not to use them during pregnancy if they have no safety data.

- Perform and record a careful risk–benefit discussion of treatment considerations (see Table 1.3).

SSRIs

- A growing literature is reporting a high incidence of serotonergic and withdrawal symptoms (including jitteriness, tremor, shivering, respiratory difficulties) in newborns exposed to SSRIs near delivery.
- Symptoms resolve in 4–5 days in most cases.

Fluoxetine (Prozac, Sarafem)

- Greatest number of reported exposures (>1,500) studied.
- Not associated with an increased risk of miscarriage or major congenital malformations.
- Neonatal complications have occurred in some cases, including jitteriness, tremor, shivering, respiratory difficulties, lower Apgar scores, special care nursery admissions.
  √ Particularly with third-trimester exposure to fluoxetine.
- Has been linked with earlier delivery (0.9-week decrease in mean gestational age in one study).
- One study reported a higher rate of multiple minor malformations in newborns exposed to fluoxetine in first trimester; subsequent studies have not reported this finding.

Citalopram (Celexa)

- Approximately 400 exposures studied.
- Not associated with an increased risk of miscarriage or major congenital malformations.
- No data available on the safety of S-citalopram (Lexapro) in pregnancy; pregnancy data from citalopram may not apply to S-citalopram.

Paroxetine (Paxil), Sertraline (Zoloft)

- Between 250–280 exposures for each studied.
- Not associated with an increased risk of miscarriage or major congenital malformations.
- Have been linked with earlier delivery (0.9-week decrease in mean gestational age in one study).
- Withdrawal and serotonergic symptoms have been reported in newborns, particularly following third-trimester use of paroxetine.
  √ Symptoms included respiratory distress, jitteriness, hypoglycemia, hypo- or hypertonia, shivering, nystagmus, and irritability.

DEPRESSIVE DISORDERS

Venlafaxine (Effexor IR, Effexor XR)

- Over 150 exposures studied.
- Not associated with an increased risk of miscarriage or major congenital malformations.

Tricyclic Antidepressants

(For example, nortriptyline [Pamelor], desipramine [Norpramin], clomipramine [Anafranil]; see Table 3.1.)

- Over 1,100 exposures (for all tricyclic antidepressants combined) studied.
- Not associated with an increased risk of miscarriage or major congenital malformations.
- Transient anticholinergic effects may occur in newborns, including constipation, tachycardia, and urinary retention.
- Perinatal toxicity or withdrawal symptoms may occur in newborns, including jitteriness, irritability, lethargy, and hypotonia.
- Among the tricyclic antidepressants, nortriptyline or desipramine should be first-line choice as each produces fewer anticholinergic and hypotensive effects.
- Blood levels of medication may need to be monitored during pregnancy, particularly if depressive symptoms recur.
- Dose may need to be increased in second and third trimesters to maintain medication blood levels within the therapeutic range.

Mirtazapine (Remeron)

- Little human data available.
- A small case series reported no perinatal complications or congenital malformations.
- Should not be used as first-line treatment of depression in pregnancy.

Bupropion (Wellbutrin IR, SR; Zyban)

- Little published data available.
- Prenatal exposure to bupropion may reduce fetal seizure threshold.
- Drug company's pregnancy registry (N = 300) shows no evidence of increased risk of birth defects.
- Should not be a first-line treatment during pregnancy.
- However, can be used for smoking cessation (either as Zyban or Wellbutrin), as the well-documented risks of nicotine exposure

during pregnancy (see Chapter 1) outweigh theoretical risk of bupropion exposure.

Nefazodone (Serzone)

- Little human data.
- Should not be used as first-line treatment for depression during pregnancy.

Monoamine Oxidase Inhibitors

(Includes isocarboxazid [Marplan]), phenelzine [Nardil], selegiline [Eldepryl], tranylcypromine [Parnate].)

- Little human data available.
- One study of 21 prenatal exposures to tranylcypromine and phenelzine reported a relative risk for congenital malformations of 3.4.
- MAOIs contraindicate the use of tocolytic agents (e.g., terbutaline), which may be necessary to prevent premature labor.
- MAOIs are best avoided in pregnant women.

Behavioral Teratogenesis Following Prenatal Exposure to Antidepressants

- Refers to the neurobehavioral sequelae in children from prenatal exposure to medications.
- The use of antidepressant during pregnancy exposes the fetal brain to psychoactive agents at a time when the central nervous system is developing.
- Medications enter fetal brains more readily than adult brains because of the relatively smaller proportion of myelin in the fetal central nervous system.
- Available (but limited) data show no difference in IQ, language development, temperament, or mood in 16–86 month-old children who were exposed to SSRIs and TCAs in utero.
- Patients should be advised of the paucity of data on long-term neurobehavioral development in children exposed to antidepressants in utero.

Electroconvulsive Therapy

- Can be safely administered during pregnancy.
- Can provide rapid stabilization of severe conditions (e.g., delusional depression, mania).

- Succinylcholine, a muscle relaxant often used during ECT, appears safe during pregnancy.
- The anticholinergic agent glycopyrrolate (to prevent bradycardia) appears safe during pregnancy and produces less fetal exposure than atropine.
- Preparation for ECT should include external fetal monitoring to rule out uterine contractions.
- External fetal monitoring should continue for several hours after ECT procedure.

Alternative Treatments

- Omega-3 fatty acids:
  - √ Promote optimal neurological and retinal development of the fetus and infant.
  - √ Appear to protect against preterm labor.
  - √ Preliminary data show omega-3 fatty acids may offer a safe alternative treatment for major depression in pregnancy and breast-feeding.
  - √ Optimal dose for treatment of depression not yet established; case reports have used 1–4 g/day of ethyl eicosapentaenoic acid (EPA) and 2 g/day of docosahexanoic acid (DHA).

Antidepressant Considerations Prior to Conception

If patient is likely to remain well off antidepressants for at least a few weeks, and she is likely to conceive quickly (i.e., she is healthy, <age 35 years, with no history of infertility in herself or her partner):

- Discontinue the antidepressant medication before she attempts to get pregnant.
- Educate the patient about ways to maximize chances of conception as quickly as possible by using methods to detect ovulation (e.g., by monitoring basal body temperature or using an OTC ovulation detection kit).

If patient is likely to remain well off antidepressants for at least a few weeks, and she is NOT likely to conceive quickly:

- Most antidepressants can be used safely while patient is *trying to conceive,* followed by quick discontinuation once pregnancy test is positive.

√ Exceptions:
  □ Venlafaxine and paroxetine, because they produce particularly severe withdrawal syndromes following abrupt discontinuation.
  □ Fluoxetine, because its long half-life produces prolonged fetal exposure after medication is discontinued.
* Continue the antidepressant medication until patient has positive pregnancy test (typically 14 days postconception, if patient performs a pregnancy test on the first day of her missed menstrual period).
* Once patient is pregnant—and if she remains euthymic—discontinue the medication.
  √ The uteroplacental circulation begins forming at approximately 2 weeks postconception.
  √ Therefore, the embryo receives minimal exposure (unless the medication has an unusually long half-life).

If patient has a history of severe relapses of depression following previous attempts at medication discontinuation:

* Continue the antidepressant during pregnancy.
* Fluoxetine, citalopram, nortriptyline are reasonable first choices (because they have the largest databases on use during pregnancy).

If patient has a history of mild or moderate relapses of depression following previous attempts at medication discontinuation:

* These cases require careful consideration.
* Make use of all available nonpharmacological interventions (e.g., psychotherapy, couples counseling).
* If nonpharmacological interventions fail, and the depression presents risks to the mother and/or fetus (e.g., poor nutrition, alcohol or nicotine use, suicidality), it is reasonable to initiate an antidepressant.
* Fluoxetine, citalopram, nortriptyline are reasonable first choices.

For all cases:

* Ensure that patients try to obtain nonpharmacological interventions (e.g., psychotherapy, couples counseling).
* These interventions may help reduce the need for pharmacological interventions.

- Some authors recommend discontinuation of the antidepressant in the 2–4 weeks prior to the estimated delivery date to minimize the risk of neonatal complications.
  - √ Increases the risk of relapse of maternal depression following delivery.

New-Onset Depression During Pregnancy

- Initiate and maximize nonpharmacological interventions (e.g., psychotherapy, couples counseling).
- Attempt to hold off use of antidepressants until at least week 12 of pregnancy.
  - √ Organogenesis mostly completed by this time.
- If antidepressant is initiated, fluoxetine, citalopram, nortriptyline are reasonable choices.
- Do not assume that medications are risk-free after the first trimester! Fetal brain continues developing throughout pregnancy.
- For severe depression (e.g., delusional depression, depression with suicidality), ECT is a reasonable option.

PHARMACOLOGICAL TREATMENT OF POSTPARTUM DEPRESSION

- Similar to nonpostpartum depression, with some exceptions:
  - √ Time to response is often longer.
  - √ Additional medications (e.g., benzodiazepines) are often necessary for anxiety, insomnia.
- For new mothers with a history of major depression, prophylaxis with an antidepressant (beginning on the first or second day after delivery) may help prevent postpartum depression.
- Estrogen for postpartum depression:
  - √ Appears to be mildly effective in the treatment and prophylaxis of postpartum depression.
    - □ However, mood-elevating effect appears significantly less robust than that of antidepressants.
  - √ Poses risks of endometrial hyperplasia and thromboembolism.
  - √ Diminishes the production of breast milk.
  - √ Further research is necessary before estrogen can be recommended in the treatment of postpartum depression.

USE OF ANTIDEPRESSANTS DURING BREAST-FEEDING

Selective Serotonin Reuptake Inhibitors
- Largest number of reported exposures (> 350) studied.
- Most consistent safety data are for paroxetine and sertraline.
- Fluoxetine also appears safe in most cases, but neonatal colic and irritability have been linked with its use in breast-feeding.
- Compared to other SSRIs, fluoxetine appears to produce greater medication exposure to nursing infants, possibly because of long half-life.

Tricyclic Antidepressants
- Nortriptyline, clomipramine, desipramine have been studied the most and appear safe to use in breast-feeding.
- Doxepin has been linked with respiratory depression in an infant and should therefore not be used by breast-feeding women.

Other Antidepressants
- Venlafaxine
  - √ The mean total medication exposure through breast milk was 6.4% of weight-adjusted maternal dose in one small case series of seven infants.
  - √ No adverse effects occurred in any of the infants.
  - √ Mothers were on 225–300 mg/day.
- Bupropion
  - √ Five reported cases of no adverse effects in the infants.
- Nefazodone
  - √ One case described drowsiness and poor feeding in a premature (36 weeks) breast-fed infant whose mother took nefazodone 300 mg/day.
- Mirtazapine
  - √ No published data on the use of mirtazapine during breast-feeding.
- These medications should probably not be used as first-line treatments for depression in nursing women because of the paucity of data regarding their safety.

Treatment Considerations for Breast-Feeding Patients Who Initiate Antidepressant Treatment
- Choose medications for which safety data exist on their use in breast-feeding.

DEPRESSIVE DISORDERS

- Prescribe the minimum dosage of medication that produces remission of symptoms.
- Consider supplementation with bottle-feeding to reduce infant's exposure.
- Nursing mothers can discard the milk with greatest medication concentration:
  - √ Peak breast milk concentrations of certain SSRIs (sertraline, fluoxetine) occur approximately 6–10 hours following maternal ingestion of the medication.
  - √ Nursing mothers can therefore pump and discard milk from this time period, to significantly reduce infant's medication exposure.
- Attempt to establish the infant's behavior, sleep and feeding patterns before beginning an antidepressant in a breast-feeding mother.
  - √ This information provides a baseline to determine whether infant experiences adverse effects (e.g., decreased appetite, increased sleepiness) from the medication exposure.
- Monitor infant following mother's initiation of antidepressant.
- Infant serum concentrations provide a measure of the infant's exposure to the medication through breast milk, but the blood draw can be traumatic to the infant, and the information is of limited value.
  - √ No cutoff has been established for a safe serum level of medication in infants.
- These serum levels need not be obtained routinely in a nursing infant.
  - √ Data may provide reassurance for some mothers, especially if the level is very low or undetectable.
- To obtain infant serum concentrations of medication:
  - √ Wait until medication serum levels are likely to be at steady state (i.e., at least five half-lives, see Table 3.8).
  - √ Ask the laboratory to use a high sensitivity assay (i.e., with limit of detection < 2 ng/ml; otherwise, assay is likely to have a limit of detection of 10–25 ng/ml).
  - √ Measure concentrations of both the parent drug and its metabolites in infant serum (see Table 3.9).
  - √ At present, no cutoff point has been established for concern over serum concentrations of antidepressant medications in infant serum.

Table 3.8. Pharmacokinetic Parameters of Certain Antidepressants

Medication	Protein Binding (%)	Half-life (hrs)
bupropion	80	21
citalopram	82	35
duloxetine	>90	12
fluoxetine	95	96–386
fluvoxamine	77	10–30
mirtazapine	85	20–40
nefazodone	99	2–5
paroxetine	93	21
S-citalopram	56	27–32
sertraline	98	26
venlafaxine	27	2–11

√ When women take standard doses of sertraline (50–200 mg/ day) or paroxetine (20–40 mg/day), medication levels in the nursing infants are typically < 10 ng/ml.

√ When women take standard doses of fluoxetine (20–40 mg/ day), fluoxetine and norfluoxetine levels in nursing infants have been higher, sometimes even at concentrations comparable to those seen in adults (i.e., 50–300 ng/ml).

√ In the absence of adverse effects in the infant, there is no reason for a woman to discontinue nursing, regardless of the infant's serum concentration.

• Infants who are premature (< 36 weeks gestation) or have hepatic dysfunction should generally not be exposed to antidepressant medications through breast milk.

• New mothers who have recently weaned their infants may experience premenstrual mood changes once menstrual cycle resumes.

• Omega-3 fatty acids may provide an alternative treatment that can be used safely during breast-feeding (see p. 56).

Table 3.9. Antidepressants and Their Metabolites

Parent Drug	Metabolite
bupropion	hydroxybupropion, threohydroxybupropion, erythrohydroxybupropion
citalopram, S-citalopram	desmethylcitalopram
fluoxetine	norfluoxetine
fluvoxamine	none
mirtazapine	desmethylmirtazapine
nefazodone	hydroxynefazodone, triazoledione and m-chlorophenylpiperazine (mCPP)
paroxetine	none
sertraline	desmethylsertraline
venlafaxine	desmethylvenlafaxine

Factors Influencing Infant's Exposure to Antidepressant Medication through Breast Milk

- Maternal dose:
  - ✓ Medications should be maintained at the lowest effective dose to miminize infant's exposure through breast milk.
- Timing of maternal dose:
  - ✓ Concentrations of some drugs are known to peak a few hours after maternal ingestion of the medication.
    - □ Sertraline and fluoxetine levels are highest 6–10 hours after the mother takes the medication.
  - ✓ However, the time when medications peak in breast milk is unknown for most medications.
- Medication properties:
  - ✓ Half-life (see Table 3.8).
    - □ Shorter half-life typically produces less exposure.
  - ✓ Protein binding (see Table 3.8).
    - □ Higher protein binding typically produces less exposure.
  - ✓ Potency.
    - □ Medications vary widely in potency (e.g., fluoxetine has approximately one-sixth and one-fifteenth the serotonergic potency of sertraline and paroxetine, respectively).
    - □ Therefore, a serum concentration of 100 ng/ml fluoxetine is approximately equivalent in potency to a serum concentration of 6.7 ng/ml paroxetine.

TREATMENT CONSIDERATIONS FOR PERI- AND POSTMENOPAUSAL WOMEN

Evaluation and Treatment of Depression

- Ask about night sweats before assuming insomnia and fatigue are secondary to depression.
  - ✓ Hormone replacement therapy (HRT) is helpful for patients with night sweats and hot flashes.
  - ✓ As night sweats and hot flashes diminish, insomnia, daytime fatigue, and mood are likely to improve.
  - ✓ Improvement typically occurs quickly, within 7–10 days.
  - ✓ If mood has not improved with HRT, initiate usual treatment for depression.
- Venlafaxine, paroxetine, and fluoxetine have been reported to significantly reduce hot flashes (independent of effects on mood).

- Women with a history of depression appear more likely to experience menopause at an earlier age.
- A risk factor for recurrent depression in older women is first-onset of depression after age 60.

Role of Estrogen

- At physiological doses (e.g., transdermal patch 100 μg; premarin 0.625–1.25 mg/day), estrogen appears to have modest mood-elevating effects and may be helpful for mild depressive symptoms.
- Effect is independent of estrogen's relief of vasomotor symptoms.
- Estrogen's efficacy for major depression, either as monotherapy or as an augmentation to antidepressants, remains inconclusive.
  √ Recent studies of estradiol for major depression have shown promising results but require replication.

TREATMENT CONSIDERATIONS FOR ELDERLY WOMEN

- See Chapter 1, pages 18–19.
- The newer antidepressants are less likely to produce medically dangerous side effects (e.g., changes in blood pressure, falls) than tricyclic antidepressants or monoamine oxidase inhibitors.
- An elderly woman experiencing cognitive deficits may benefit from an evaluation for depression.
  √ If she is depressed and receives treatment, cognitive functioning may subsequently improve.
- Treatment noncompliance is a particular challenge in the treatment of elderly patients because they may forget when to take their medication or confuse one medication with another.

TREATMENT-RESISTANT DEPRESSION

- Patients who do not respond to two full trials of antidepressants are considered treatment-resistant.
- Surprisingly few controlled studies have systematically examined approaches to treatment-resistant patients.
- Even fewer studies have examined comparative approaches to antidepressant treatment failures.

Table 3.10. Approaches to Treatment-Resistant Depression

First Line	Second Line	Other Treatments
Lithium	Buspirone	Estrogen
T3	Atypical neuroleptic	Anticonvulsants
Combination of antidepressants		DHEA
Stimulants		Light therapy
		Pindolol

Approaches to Treatment-Resistant Depression

- Review diagnosis.
- Screen for comorbid diagnoses that may affect treatment response, either medical (e.g., hypothyroidism) or psychiatric (especially drug/alcohol abuse).
- Review treatment adherence.
- Specific approaches to treatment resistant depression are listed in Table 3.10.

Pharmacological Approaches

- Optimization:
  √ Use the original antidepressant for longer than 6 weeks or at higher than usual dose.
- Switching:
  √ To another antidepressant, either within the same class (e.g., a second SSRI) or across antidepressant classes.
  √ If patient has failed two agents within the same class (e.g., two SSRIs), switch class of antidepressant.
- Augmentation:
  √ Add a second agent (e.g., lithium, methylphenidate) that augments the effect of the antidepressant.
- Combination:
  √ Add a second agent that is also an antidepressant (typically with different neurotransmitter effects than the original agent).
- Lithium:
  √ Most well-documented approach.
  √ Nevertheless, infrequently used because of side effects, need for blood tests.
  √ Prescribe 900 mg/day (or 300–600 mg/day in patients over 65 years).
  √ Trial takes 2–3 weeks.

√ Serum lithium levels are less relevant than for bipolar disorder (but should be monitored to avoid toxicity).
- Triiodothyronine (T3; Cytomel), a thyroid hormone:
  √ Benign and occasionally effective.
  √ May also help accelerate response to antidepressants, particularly in women.
  √ Typically prescribed at 25–37.5 μg/day.
  √ Higher doses may promote bone loss and should be used with caution in women at risk for osteoporosis (e.g., smokers; family history of osteoporosis).
  √ Trial takes 3 weeks.
  √ Pretreatment thyroid indices do not predict response.
- Combination of antidepressants:
  √ Virtually no studies have examined combination treatment, but this approach is popular among clinicians.
  √ Can combine any two antidepressants, except: Do not combine MAOIs with SSRIs, venlafaxine, bupropion, duloxetine, nefazodone, mirtazapine, or clomipramine.
  √ If combining tricyclic with MAOI, add MAOI to tricyclic (not vice versa).
  √ Most common combination is SSRI or venlafaxine with bupropion (since there is little overlap in neurotransmitter effect between the two agents).
  √ Optimal dosing is unclear (i.e., use full doses of both agents vs. lower doses of one or the other).
  √ If combining tricyclic with either fluoxetine or paroxetine, use lower doses of the tricyclic (as fluoxetine and paroxetine may inhibit its metabolism) and monitor tricyclic blood level.
- Stimulants (see below):
  √ Very popular with many clinicians, despite lack of controlled data supporting use.
  √ Used safely with all antidepressants except MAOIs.
  √ Can be used with MAOIs but with great caution regarding drug–drug interactions.
  √ All stimulants appear equally effective.
  √ When effective, they work quickly (i.e., within days).
- Buspirone:
  √ Typically used mostly with anxious patients.
  √ Unclear efficacy.
  √ Usually prescribed at 20–60 mg/day, but optimal doses are unclear.

- Atypical neuroleptics:
  - √ Supported by one controlled study and much clinical experience.
  - √ Probably all atypical neuroleptics are equally effective, but risperidone and olanzapine have been most commonly prescribed.
  - √ Optimal doses are unclear.
    - □ Most clinicians use low doses (e.g., risperidone 0.5–3 mg/day; olanzapine 2.5–10 mg/day).
  - √ Timing of effect is variable, from days to weeks.
- Estrogen:
  - √ For more information about using estrogen for depression, see p. 63.

Stimulants
- Biological effects:
  - √ Increase dopamine through direct release and reuptake blockade.
  - √ Similar, less consistent effects on norepinephrine.
- Clinical effects:
  - √ Primary effects are to increase arousal and attention.
  - √ Secondary, less consistent, effects are to improve mood.
  - √ Also used to reduce appetite.
  - √ Effects are immediate regardless of clinical indication.
  - √ Clinical activity is apparent within hours to days.
- First-line agents:
  - √ Methylphenidate and d-amphetamine, in various preparations (see Table 3.11).
  - √ Preparations differ primarily by half-life and are prescribed either once daily (long half-life agents) or up to qid (short half-life agents).

Less commonly prescribed stimulants are listed in Table 3.12.

- New stimulants:
  - √ Modafinil (Provigil).
    - □ Once daily dosing.
    - □ Dosage listed in Table 3.12.
    - □ May be more effective for energy than attention/concentration.
    - □ Nontriplicate.

Table 3.11. Available Preparations of Methylphenidate and D-Amphetamine

Preparation	Brand Names	Dosage (mg)	Duration of Action (hrs)
methylphenidate	Ritalin, Methylin	20–80	3½–4
	Focalin	10–40	4
	Ritalin-SR	20–80	3–6
	Ritalin LA	20–80	7–8
	Metadate CD	20–80	7–8
	Concerta	18–90	8–10
d-amphetamine	Dexedrine, Dextrostat	10–60	4
	Dexedrine spansules	10–60	5–6
	Adderall	10–60	5–6
	Adderall XR	10–60	8–11

√ Atomoxetine (Strattera).

- Selective norepinephrine reuptake inhibitor.
- Once daily dosing in A.M.
- Full dose 1–1.2 mg/kg/day.
- Taken after meals.
- Nontriplicate.

Potential Side Effects

- Side effects that may occur with all stimulants include:

√ Anxiety.

√ Irritability.

√ Insomnia.

√ Headache.

√ Decreased appetite.

√ Weight loss (initially).

√ Mild tachycardia.

- Atomoxetine—potential additional side effects:

√ Dry mouth.

√ Dizziness.

Table 3.12. Available Preparations of Alternative Stimulants

Preparation	Brand Name	Dosage (mg)
d-methamphetamine	Desoxyn	5–40
pemoline	Cylert	18.75–150
phentermine	Ionamin	15–30
	Fastin	15–30
diethylpropion	Tenuate	25–100
phendimetrazine	Plegine, Prelu-2	35–105
modafinil	Provigil	100–400
atomoxetine	Strattera	40–100

√ Urinary hesitation.
√ Nausea.
- Pemoline—potential additional side effects:
  √ Associated with hepatoxicity.
  √ Rarely used currently.

Potential for Abuse/Dependence
- Uncommon.
- Use with caution in patients with a history of stimulant abuse or eating disorders.

Use of Stimulants during Pregnancy and Breast-Feeding
- Most data involve prenatal exposure to amphetamines, much of it drawn from studies of maternal amphetamine abuse.
- Prenatal amphetamine exposure does not appear to produce fetal congenital malformations.
- Less information is available about prenatal exposure to methylphenidate.
  √ Available data do not show evidence of teratogenicity.
- Maternal abuse of amphetamines during pregnancy is linked with
  √ Intrauterine growth retardation.
  √ Premature delivery.
  √ Withdrawal symptoms in newborns.
- Little is known about the safety of stimulants during breast-feeding—therefore, stimulants are best avoided by nursing women.

Electroconvulsive Therapy

- Used with:
  √ Treatment-refractory patients.
  √ Patients in clinically urgent situations (e.g., with escalating suicidality).
  √ Patients with psychotic features.
- At least as effective as antidepressants.
- Can be used with inpatients or outpatients (the latter require someone to drive them home after treatment).
- Typical course is 6–12 treatments, administered 2–3 times weekly.
- Important technical variables affecting both efficacy and side effects include:
  √ Voltage.
  √ Lead placement (e.g., unilateral vs. bilateral)

- Presence of electrical seizure (manifestations blocked by succin-lycholine, a short-acting muscle paralyzing agent) necessary but not sufficient for efficacy.
- Side effects
  - √ Headache after each treatment: benign, relatively easily treated.
  - √ Cognitive effects: posttreatment confusion, increasing with each treatment.
  - √ Anterograde and retrograde amnesia, maximal around the time of ECT; otherwise, memory deficits are transient in most patients.
  - √ Medically serious side effects are now extremely rare.
- Use of medications with ECT:
  - √ Avoid lithium (exacerbates confusion).
  - √ Avoid anticonvulsants and benzodiazepines (increase seizure threshold).
  - √ Can use trazodone for sleep.
  - √ Antidepressants (except MAOIs) and antipsychotics pose no problems.
- Continuation/maintenance ECT:
  - √ Antidepressants are frequently ineffective in preventing recurrence of depression after effective ECT.
  - √ Maintenance ECT is an alternative to antidepressants; involves gradually tapering treatments to once monthly.

DEPRESSIVE DISORDERS

4. Bipolar Disorder

The prevalence of bipolar disorder is approximately equal among men and women. However, gender differences arise in the symptoms and clinical course of the illness. Women with bipolar disorder are more likely than men to experience recurrent depressive episodes, and some studies show that women are more likely to follow a rapid-cycling course (i.e. > four mood episodes/year). The greater incidence of rapid cycling among female patients may reflect their greater incidence of depression and use of antidepressants. The depressions of bipolar disorder are characterized by the same range of symptoms as classic major depression, but hypersomnia, hyperphagia, and psychomotor retardation are relatively more common in bipolar depression.

The course of bipolar disorder may vary at different times in women's reproductive lives. Premenstrually, symptoms may recur or worsen, and serum lithium levels may drop in women who experience marked premenstrual edema. Some studies have reported that the risk of relapse of bipolar disorder is reduced during pregnancy, whereas others show no change in the course of the illness. However, women with bipolar disorder face an unequivocal risk of relapse following delivery. The relapse can manifest as either a depressive or manic episode. Patients also may present with postpartum psychosis, a poorly defined syndrome with features resembling both mania and delirium. In many, if not most, cases postpartum psychosis appears to represent a manifestation of bipolar or schizoaffective disorder. The precise diagnostic criteria for postpartum psychosis remain to be defined. It is not included as a discrete diagnosis in *Diagnostic and Statistical*

BIPOLAR DISORDER

Manual-IV (*DSM-IV*) but instead is described through the use of the "postpartum-onset" specifier, which is applied to a manic episode, brief psychotic disorder, or psychosis not otherwise specified.

Because bipolar disorder is virtually always recurrent, long-term maintenance treatment is an integral part of the overall treatment plan. Although the consensus of the field is to seriously consider maintenance treatment after even a single manic episode (since future episodes are highly likely), it is often exceedingly difficult to convince young persons to agree to extended, probably lifetime, treatment without having a second episode to persuade them of the recurrent nature of bipolar disorder.

Women who decide to remain on mood stabilizers indefinitely may face challenges in their family-planning decisions. Fears of the teratogenic effects of mood stabilizers and of a potential relapse of illness during pregnancy lead some women with bipolar disorder to avoid pregnancy. Information on approaches to minimize risks to the mother and fetus during pregnancy is not easily accessible for large numbers of patients.

Patients with bipolar disorder often face challenges in their roles as parents. Their dramatic mood, behavior, and personality changes can bewilder and frighten their children. Clinicians should emphasize that stability and treatment compliance are important not only for patients but also for the well-being of their children. Patients should be encouraged to identify family members or friends to whom they can turn for help with child-care responsibilities during future relapses when planning for the illness.

Most research studies of bipolar disorder have focused on bipolar I disorder; much less is known about bipolar II disorder. Available literature shows that bipolar II disorder appears to occur more commonly in women than men. The course of bipolar II disorder has not been well established, but it appears to be distinct: bipolar II disorder does *not* generally evolve into bipolar I disorder. The overall treatment strategy for bipolar II disorder is similar to bipolar I disorder, although mood stabilizers are less essential. Clinicians may prescribe antidepressants alone (i.e., without a mood stabilizer) to some bipolar II patients, because even if the patients switch into a hypomanic state (a known risk from all antidepressants given to bipolar patients), the severity of the switch is significantly less (hypomanic episodes are, by definition, milder than manic episodes). Clinicians should be careful to distinguish bipolar II from PMDD, another cyclic disorder character-ized by abrupt changes in mood (see Chapter 7).

Recently, the boundaries of bipolar disorder have been expanded by some experts to include patients with subtler mood swings—e.g., hy-pomanic episodes lasting less than the 4 days required by the *DSM-IV*. Distinguishing these milder "bipolar spectrum" disorders from the mood instability associated with certain personality disorders is clinically difficult. Compounding the diagnostic challenge, patients frequently exhibit bipolar spectrum syndromes in addition to the af-fective instability associated with personality disorders. In these cir-cumstances, diagnostic precision is almost impossible.

Comorbid alcohol and substance use disorders also complicate the di-agnosis of bipolar disorder. Approximately 20% of female and 40–50% of male patients with bipolar disorder suffer from comorbid alcohol and substance use disorders. Untreated, these comorbidities predict significantly worse treatment outcomes.

MOOD STABILIZERS/ANTIMANIC AGENTS

Table 4.1 lists mood stabilizers and their efficacy for the different phases of bipolar disorder.

Valproate (Depakote, Depakote-ER, Depakene)

* Most commonly prescribed mood stabilizer in the United States, due to documented efficacy, patient acceptance, and aggressive marketing.

Table 4.1. Efficacy of Mood Stabilizers for Bipolar Disorder

Generic Name (Brand Name)	Acute Mania	Maintenance	Acute Depression
valproate (Depakene, Depakote, Depakote-ER)	++	++	?+
lithium (Eskalith, Eskalith CR Lithobid)	++	++	+
carbamazepine (Tegretol)	+	+	0-?
lamotrigine (Lamictal)	0-?	++	++
olanzapine (Zyprexa)	++	++	?-+
gabapentin (Neurontin)	0-?	0-?	0-?
topiramate (Topamax)	0-?	?	?
oxcarbazepine (Trileptal)	+	?+	?
clozapine (Clozaril)	++	++	?+
ECT	++	+	++

0 = no efficacy; 0-? = possible efficacy; + = some efficacy; ++ = substantial efficacy

- Available as antiepileptic drug for over 20 years.
- Acute antimanic efficacy data:
  - √ Strong and consistent.
  - √ Equivalent to lithium.
  - √ Better tolerated than lithium.
- Patients gradually improve over 3–6 weeks.
  - √ Over first 3 weeks, fewer than half will improve substantially.
- Acute antidepressant efficacy data:
  - √ Inconsistent evidence of efficacy.
- Maintenance treatment data:
  - √ Generally considered effective against both mania and depression, despite only modest evidence.

Pretreatment Workup
- Before initiating valproate, obtain:
  - √ Complete blood count, including platelets.
  - √ Chemistry panel, including liver function tests.
  - √ β-HCG (in reproductive-aged women).

Dosing
- Typical doses: 750–3000 mg/day.
- Average dose for acute mania: 1500–2000 mg/day.
- Available as:
  - √ Generic valproate.
  - √ Depakene.
  - √ Depakote (trade name; enteric coated, with fewer GI side effects).
  - √ Depakote-ER (trade name; extended release, which requires 15%–20% higher doses than Depakote or generic valproate due to decreased absorption).
- For inpatients, two titration schedules:
  - √ Start at 250 mg tid or 500 mg bid and increase by 250 mg/day as tolerated.
  - √ Start at 20 mg/kg/day in divided doses.
    - □ Obtain valproate level in 2–3 days and adjust dose for desired level.
    - □ May yield quicker improvement but requires more careful monitoring and has greater initial side effects.
- For outpatients, start 250 mg bid or tid and gradually increase as tolerated.
- Target serum level: 50–100 mcg/ml.

- Some patients may need serum level up to 125 mcg/ml.
- Initial dose for inpatients administered in divided doses.
- Outpatients may be treated with once daily (typically evening) dosing from treatment onset.

Potential Side Effects
- Nausea.
- Tremor.
- Sedation.
- Weight gain.
- Hair loss.
- Menstrual disturbances.
- Hyperandrogenism.
- Polycystic ovary syndrome (PCOS; see below)
  - √ Believed to result from valproate-induced hyperinsulinemia.
  - √ Elevated insulin levels inhibit conversion of testosterone to estradiol, producing the hyperandrogenic state that leads to menstrual irregularities and PCOS.
  - √ Young women (< 20 years) appear to be particularly at risk.
  - √ Valproate-induced PCOS may reverse with time (> 3 years) on valproate.
- Reduction of bone-mineral density and increased risk of bone fractures:
  - √ Mechanisms are unclear but may involve inhibition of parathyroid hormone or increased metabolism of vitamin D.
  - √ In women at risk for osteoporosis (e.g., family history of osteoporosis; long-term nicotine use), valproate may not be ideal first-line agent.
- Hepatitis (or marked increase in transaminase levels)—rare.
- Pancreatitis—rare.
- Thrombocytopenia—rare.

Polycystic Ovary Syndrome (PCOS)

√ Affects approximately 7% of women of reproductive age.
√ Most common cause of infertility.
√ Increases risk of diabetes, heart disease, endometrial cancer.
√ Signs and symptoms:
  □ Hirsutism.
  □ Obesity.
  □ Acne.

    □ Elevated androgens and luteinizing hormone.
    □ Chronic anovulation.
    □ Insulin resistance.

Treatment of Specific Side Effects
* Nausea:
    √ Use the enteric-coated or extended-release formulation of valproate (i.e., Depakote or depakote-ER).
    √ Use H-2 blockers (e.g., Zantac, Tagamet, Pepcid).
* Polycystic ovary syndrome:
    √ Begin an oral contraceptive.
        □ Yasmin is a good choice because it contains a novel progestin (drospirenone) with antiandrogenic properties.
    √ Use an insulin sensitizer.
        □ These help correct the insulin resistance that occurs with PCOS, subsequently reducing androgen levels and restoring ovulation.
        □ They include:
            Glucophage (metformin).
            Avandia (rosiglitazone).
            Actos (pioglitazone).

Blood Monitoring
* Clinicians often obtain CBC and liver function tests every few months with patients on valproate:
    √ The utility of these tests is unclear.
* Occasional monitoring of valproate levels (e.g., at 6-month intervals) may help in ensuring adequate dosing.
* For female patients, obtain:
    √ Serum testosterone, androstenedione, if evidence of hyperandrogenism, (acne, weight gain, hirsutism, male-pattern hair loss [e.g., receding hairline in temporal area of forehead]).
    √ β-HCG in reproductive-aged women who miss a menstrual period or have had recent unprotected intercourse.

Recommended Monitoring for Women of Reproductive Age on Valproate
* Monitor for changes in menstrual pattern.
* Monitor for evidence of hyperandrogenism (acne, weight gain, hirsutism, male-pattern hair loss [e.g., receding hairline in temporal area of forehead]).

Lithium (Lithobid, Eskalith, Eskalith-CR)

- Oldest mood stabilizer available.
- Supplanted by valproate as most commonly prescribed mood stabilizer in the United States.
- Remains the dominant mood stabilizer in many other countries.
- Is not metabolized by liver; excreted by kidneys.
  √ Excretion varies with glomerular filtration rate.
  √ Increases during pregnancy, decreases among elderly.
- Reaches steady state in 4–5 days.
- Clear efficacy in preventing manic episodes, but little recent consistent efficacy in preventing depressions.
- Predictors of good response:
  √ Euphoric (classic) mania.
    □ Lithium is less effective than valproate or atypical antipsychotics for mixed states.
  √ Sequence of mania followed by depression.
  √ No psychosis.
  √ No rapid cycling.

Pretreatment Workup
- Tests of renal function (e.g., serum creatinine).
- TSH.
- For patients over age 40, consider obtaining EKG.
- β-HCG (in reproductive-aged women).

Dosing
- Lithium is available as:
  √ Lithium carbonate.
  √ Lithobid (slow-release formulation).
  √ Eskalith.
  √ Eskalith-CR (slow-release formulation).
- Slow-release formulations produce less nausea in beginning of treatment; few differences thereafter.
- For acute inpatient mania:
  √ Starting daily dose:
    □ 900 mg/day, in divided doses, for young adults.
    □ 600 mg/day for older adults (age 40–60).
    □ 300 mg/day for adults over 65.
- For outpatients:
  √ Starting daily dose: 300 mg bid.

BIPOLAR DISORDER

√ Check lithium level in 5 days.
√ Gradually increase dose to achieve desired level.
- After dose stabilization, patients may take entire dose once daily, if desired.

Lithium Levels
- Lithium dose is regulated by serum levels more than any other psychotropic medication.
- Lithium levels should be drawn 12 hours (10–14 hours) after the last lithium dose.
- Fasting is not required prior to lithium level.
- If patient is taking entire daily lithium dose once daily, keep in mind that blood levels will be 25% higher than if patient were taking the same dose bid or tid.
- For acute mania, optimal plasma level: 0.8–1.2 mEq/l; for geriatric patients, 0.4–0.8 mEq/l.
- For maintenance treatment, optimal plasma level: 0.5–1.0 mEq/l; for geriatric patients, 0.3–0.8 mEq/l.
- Check serum level within a few days after initiating treatment and adjust dose according to target level.
- Steady-state levels are reached in 4–5 days but in inpatient setting, need for approximate values dominates.
  √ Obtain level as early as 2 days after starting lithium.

Potential Side Effects
- Polyuria.
- Polydipsia.
- Weight gain.
- Tremor.
- Cognitive impairment (e.g., impaired memory, decreased creativity, decreased concentration).
- Nausea (usually early in treatment).
- Acne.
- Hair loss—rare.
- Irregular menses—rare; secondary to hypothyroidism (see Table 1.2).

Treatment of Specific Side Effects
- Nausea:
  √ Switch to sustained-release agent and dose immediately after meals.

- Tremor:
  - √ Use beta-blockers (e.g., propanolol 10–20 mg bid–qid).
- Polyuria, polydipsia:
  - √ Use diuretics:
    - □ Caution re: hypotension.
    - □ Caution re: lithium levels, which can become toxic with use of diuretics.
    - □ Can use potassium-sparing diuretics:
      - Amiloride 5–10 mg/day.
      - Triamterene 100–300 mg/day.
    - □ Can use thiazide diuretics (e.g., hydrochlorothiazide 12.5–50 mg/day) but check potassium and add potassium supplements as necessary.
- Weight gain:
  - √ Add topiramate 50–100 mg/day (see p. 87).
- Acne:
  - √ Use benzoyl peroxide topical cream and/or antibiotics (e.g., minocycline 75 mg/day).

Potential Organ Toxicity
- Thyroid (hypothyroidism):
  - √ Progressive, correlates with time on lithium.
  - √ Risk for women is much higher than for men.
    - □ Possibly due to women's higher likelihood of having preexisting antithyroid antibodies.
  - √ Treat by administration of thyroid hormone supplementation
    - □ L-thyroxine, typical dose: 25–150 mcg/day.
  - √ After initiating thyroid supplementation, check thyroid function (i.e., TSH) approximately 6 weeks later.
  - √ Subsequently adjust thyroid supplementation, as necessary, to achieve TSH within normal range.
  - √ Hypothyroidism is *not* a justification for lithium discontinuation.
- Kidneys:
  - √ 10–20% of patients exposed to > 10 years of lithium develop interstitial nephritis.
  - √ Tubular dysfunction, characterized by nephrogenic diabetes insipidus, is an early symptom.
  - √ Later signs include a rising serum creatinine.
  - √ If serum creatinine > 1.5 mg/dl, obtain renal consultation and consider switching to another mood stabilizer.

BIPOLAR DISORDER

- Skin:
  √ Exacerbation of psoriasis.
- Parathyroid gland:
  √ Hyperparathyroidism, with subsequent elevation of serum calcium.
  √ Associated with fatigue, muscle aches, cognitive impairment, apathy, abdominal distress, loss of appetite, osteoporosis, and osteopenia.
- Cardiovascular:
  √ T-wave flattening or inversion—benign.
  √ Sinus node dysfunction—rare.

Lithium Intoxication
- Can occur when serum levels exceed 1.3 mEq/l.
- May be serious or even fatal.
- Signs/symptoms:
  √ Worsening tremor.
  √ Vomiting.
  √ Diarrhea.
  √ Ataxia.
  √ Slurred speech.
  √ Confusion.
- If suspected, discontinue lithium and obtain immediate blood level.
- Consider medical hospitalization.

Blood Monitoring
- Obtain every 6–12 months:
  √ Creatinine.
  √ TSH.
- If patient reports symptoms suggestive of hypothyroidism, obtain thyroid test sooner:
  √ Women > 40 years are particularly at risk for thyroid dysfunction.
  √ Symptoms of hypothyroidism are listed in Table 1.2.
- Check lithium level every 4–6 months in stable patients maintained on unchanging dose.
- If lithium dose is adjusted or a medication is added that may alter lithium levels (e.g., NSAIDS, diuretic), check lithium level 5 days later.
- Lithium levels are altered by hydration status (e.g., hot days, fasting, diarrhea, fever, change in salt or caffeine intake, diuretic use).

Female-Specific Considerations in Using Lithium

- NSAIDs reduce lithium clearance and can produce lithium toxicity.
  - √ Warn women on lithium not to use NSAIDs for premenstrual cramping.
- Several diuretics reduce lithium clearance and can produce lithium toxicity.
  - √ Warn women on lithium not to use diuretics for premenstrual bloating (especially thiazide diuretics, as these are most likely to increase lithium levels).
- Lithium should not be a first-line agent in patients with active eating disorders who engage in frequent purging and use laxatives and diuretics.
  - √ If lithium is used in these patients, lithium levels should be followed closely.
- Women are more likely than men to suffer from autoimmune illnesses (e.g., psoriasis, systemic lupus erythematosus) and lithium's immuno-stimulating properties may exacerbate or activate such illnesses.
- Lithium may theoretically increase the risk for osteoporosis because of hyperparathyroidism risk and subsequent loss of bone calcification.
  - √ In the absence of hyperparathyroidism, lithium does not pose such risk.

Carbamazepine (Tegretol)

- First antiepileptic drug used to treat bipolar disorder in late 1970s and early 1980s.
- Used less today than previously because of side-effect profile, compared to other agents, and loss of patent (leading to less research and less promotion).
- Data supporting its efficacy are less clear than for valproate and lithium.
- Carbamazepine's use is typically limited by its side effects.
- For acute mania:
  - √ Probably equivalent to lithium.
  - √ In one study, demonstrated less efficacy compared to valproate.
- For acute depression, little is known about carbamazepine's efficacy.

- For maintenance treatment, data supporting its efficacy are inconsistent.

Pretreatment Workup
- Before initiating treatment, obtain:
  - √ CBC with differential.
  - √ Chemistry panel, including serum sodium and liver function tests.
  - √ β-HCG (in reproductive-aged women).
- In patient's medical history, look for evidence of drug-induced blood dyscrasias.
  - √ Best not to use carbamazepine in patients with previous drug-induced blood dyscrasias.

Dosing
- Typical doses: 400–1800 mg/day.
- For acute inpatient mania:
  - √ Start with 200 mg bid (or tid, if the patient has tolerated carbamazepine well in the past).
  - √ Increase by 200 mg every 1–2 days, as tolerated.
- For outpatient hypomania and for maintenance treatment:
  - √ Begin 100 mg bid or 200 mg in evening.
  - √ Increase by 100–200 mg every few days, as tolerated.
- Prescribe in divided doses—bid or tid—to minimize side effects.
  - √ Can be prescribed once daily, if patient tolerates it.

Potential Side Effects
- Ataxia.
- Fatigue.
- Psychomotor incoordination.
- Double vision.
- Benign rash—not dose related.
- Hyponatremia—not dose related:
  - √ Characterized in early stages by lethargy and "spaciness."
  - √ Relatively common side effect in older patients.
- Benign leukopenia:
  - √ Responds to dose reduction.
  - √ Not related to more severe blood dyscrasias (described in following points).

- Agranulocytosis, aplastic anemia:
  - √ Rare.
  - √ Occurs most commonly in first 6 months of treatment, but possible thereafter.
  - √ Almost impossible to predict by routine CBCs.
  - √ Instruct patients to call if infection, fever, or easy bruising/ bleeding and obtain immediate CBC.
- Severe rash (Stevens–Johnson syndrome/toxic epidermal necrolysis):
  - √ Rare.
  - √ Severe, widespread, vesicular formation, mucosal involvement, likely to be preceded by fever and pharyngitis.
- Reduction in bone-mineral density and increased risk of bone fractures (similar to valproate, see p. 75).

Drug Interactions
- Carbamazepine induces the metabolism of many medications, including:
  - √ Itself.
  - √ Other antiepileptic drugs.
  - √ Antipsychotic agents.
  - √ Antidepressants.
  - √ Oral contraceptives (see p. 26).
  - √ Protease inhibitors.
- If patients are on any of these medications when they begin carbamazepine, be aware of potential changes in blood levels.
  - √ Check levels and adjust doses, as clinically indicated.

Blood Monitoring
- Routine CBCs are typically obtained, especially complete blood count, every 2–4 weeks during first 6 months.
  - √ Liver function tests every 2–3 months for the first 6 months, thereafter, every 6 months (at most).
- Serum levels of carbamazepine:
  - √ Typical levels are 4–12 mcg/ml.
  - √ Levels do not correlate with efficacy.
  - √ Use as guideline only.
- Because carbamazepine induces its own metabolism, its serum level (and possibly its effect) diminishes 2–4 weeks after beginning treatment.

B
I
P
O
L
A
R

D
I
S
O
R
D
E
R

Lamotrigine (Lamictal)

- Antiepileptic drug used increasingly over the last few years, especially for bipolar depression.
- For acute mania:
  √ Weak evidence of efficacy.
  √ Lamotrigine's required slow titration schedule significantly limits its use for mania.
- For acute depression:
  √ Clear evidence of efficacy in most studies.
- For maintenance treatment:
  √ Effective in preventing depressions.
  √ Efficacy in preventing mania is less consistent.
- May help delay episodes in rapid-cycling bipolar II patients, but not bipolar I patients.
- For treatment-refractory bipolar disorder, preliminary data show lamotrigine may be less effective for women than men.

Pretreatment Workup
- β-HCG (in reproductive-aged women).
- No additional pretreatment labs necessary.

Dosing
- Usual dose range: 50–500 mg/day.
- Usually administered bid, but can be prescribed once daily.
- To avoid serious, potentially life-threatening rash, lamotrigine requires a slow dose titration.
- When prescribed without other antiepileptic drugs:
  √ 25 mg/day for 2 weeks.
  √ Then 50 mg/day for 2 weeks.
  √ Then increase by 50 mg weekly.
- When prescribed with valproate, halve the schedule:
  √ 12.5 mg/day (or 25 mg every other day) for 2 weeks.
  √ Then 25 mg/day for 2 weeks.
  √ Then increase by 25 mg weekly.
- When prescribed with carbamazepine, double the schedule:
  √ 50 mg/day for 2 weeks.
  √ Then 100 mg/day for 2 weeks.
  √ Then increase by 100 mg weekly.
- Dose titration is the same for inpatients and outpatients.

Potential Side Effects
- Dizziness.
- Nausea.
- Ataxia.
- Dry mouth.
- Sedation (mild compared to other antiepileptic drug mood stabilizers).
- Benign rash (unrelated to serious rash.)
- Serious rash: Stevens–Johnson syndrome/toxic epidermal necrolysis:
  - √ Rare.
  - √ Incidence 0.3% in early studies, using more aggressive dosing schedule.
  - √ Incidence in recent studies 1/6,000, probably due to slower dose titration.
  - √ Increased risk of rash associated with faster dose titration and concomitant use of valproate (since it raises lamotrigine blood levels, requiring the slower dose titration described above).
  - √ Rash typically (but not always) occurs within the first 8 weeks of treatment.
  - √ Hallmark of serious rash: severe, widespread, vesicular formation, mucosal involvement, likely to be preceded by fever and pharyngitis.

Blood Monitoring
- No need for blood monitoring.

Olanzapine

- Of the atypical antipsychotic agents, olanzapine has the best documentation of efficacy for bipolar disorder.
- Acute antimanic efficacy is well established.
- Also appears effective as adjunct to lithium or valproate.
- For bipolar depression, preliminary data show efficacy as adjunct to antidepressant.
- As maintenance treatment, preliminary data also show olanzapine may be effective as monotherapy or as adjunctive treatment.

Pretreatment Workup
- β-HCG (in reproductive-aged women).
- No additional pretreatment labs necessary.

Dosing
- Dose range: 5–30 mg/day (similar to doses for treatment of schizophrenia).
- For treating inpatient mania, start at 10–15 mg/day.
- Some patients may require up to 30 mg/day.
- No data are available on the relative efficacy of high dose vs. usual dose.
- For outpatient mania, start with 5–10 mg daily.
  √ May increase dose if side effects are not problematic.
- May be prescribed either once daily (typically at night) or in divided dose regimen for therapeutic use of sedation.

Potential Side Effects

See p. 137.

Other Atypical Antipsychotic Agents

Risperidone, quetiapine, ziprasidone also appear effective for acute mania. (See Chapter 6 for dose titration and side-effect details.)

Gabapentin (Neurontin)

- Antiepileptic drug, commonly used in inpatient and outpatient settings to decrease arousal and anxiety.
- Generally well tolerated.
- No evidence of efficacy for bipolar disorder.
- Nonetheless, prescribed frequently by clinicians as sole or adjunctive treatment for mania, depression, or maintenance treatment.

Pretreatment Workup
- β-HCG (in reproductive-aged women).
- No additional pretreatment labs necessary.

Dosing
- Because gabapentin is not metabolized but renally excreted, check renal function (serum creatinine) before treatment, if there are any reasons to suspect renal problems.
- Dose range: 600–4800 mg/day; typical doses: 1200–2400 mg/day
- For acute mania, start with 300 mg tid and increase as needed.
- Typically prescribed in divided doses because of short half-life.
- Do not prescribe > 1200 mg at one dose, secondary to limited absorption capacity.

Potential Side Effects
- Somnolence.
- Dizziness/ataxia.

Blood Monitoring
- No need for blood monitoring.

Topiramate (Topamax)

- An antiepileptic drug.
- Recently popular because it promotes weight loss.
- So far, does not appear particularly effective for bipolar disorder.

Pretreatment Workup
- Before prescribing topiramate, obtain history of renal problems.
  √ Topiramate predisposes to renal stones.
- β-HCG (in reproductive-aged women).
- No additional pretreatment labs necessary.

Dosing
- Dose range: 100–600 mg/day.
- Typical dose: 150–400 mg/day.
- Start with 25–50 mg/day; increase by 25–50 mg every 3–5 days.
- Usually prescribed bid.

Potential Side Effects
- Somnolence.
- Dizziness.
- Weight loss.
- Cognitive impairment:
  √ Ranges from word-finding difficulties to poor memory to confusion.
  √ Can be very distressing, but is completely reversible upon medication discontinuation.
- Renal stones—rare.

Blood Monitoring
- No need for blood monitoring.

B
I
P
O
L
A
R

D
I
S
O
R
D
E
R

Oxcarbazepine (Trileptal)

- An analog of carbamazepine.
- Fewer side effects than carbamazepine, so often prescribed in its stead.
- Limited data demonstrate potential efficacy in acute mania.
- Given similar efficacy to carbamazepine in epilepsy, clinicians assume equal efficacy in bipolar disorder.

Pretreatment Workup
- β-HCG (in reproductive-aged women).
- No additional pretreatment labs necessary.

Dosing
- Equivalent doses are 150% higher than carbamazepine.
  - √ Therefore, 100 mg carbamazepine = 150 mg oxcarbazepine, etc.
- Dosing strategies are similar to carbamazepine (see p. 82):
  - √ For inpatient mania, start with 300 mg bid and increase by 300 mg every few days, as tolerated, to typical doses of 600–2400 mg/day.
  - √ For outpatients, start with 300 mg at bedtime and increase by 150–300 mg every few days, as tolerated.
- Usually prescribed in divided dose regimen, like carbamazepine.

Potential Side Effects
- Similar to carbamazepine, except:
  - √ No blood dyscrasias (agranulocytosis, aplastic anemia).
  - √ Lesser intensity of typical side effects (ataxia, diplopia, etc.).
  - √ Same or greater rate of hyponatremia.
  - √ Fewer pharmacokinetic effects, except for oral contraceptives, which may be ineffective when coprescribed.

Blood Monitoring
- No need for blood monitoring.

Clozapine (Clozaril)

- Generally considered very useful for treatment-resistant bipolar disorder.
- Details on its use and side effects are described in Chapter 5 (pp. 141–142).

Benzodiazepines

- Often prescribed adjunctively in treating acute mania/hypomania.
  √ Generally helpful in promoting sleep and decreasing arousal.
- No evidence of efficacy as maintenance treatment.
- Clonazepam and lorazepam most commonly used.

Dosing
- Typically prescribed at higher doses than for treatment of anxiety.
- Starting doses: clonazepam 1 mg bid–tid; lorazepam 2 mg tid.
  √ Can increase, as needed, to clonazepam 6–8 mg/day; lorazepam 8–12 mg/day.

Potential Side Effects

See Chapter 5 (pp. 113–115).

Electroconvulsive Therapy (ECT)

- A few small controlled studies and much anecdotal data demonstrate its efficacy in acute mania.
- Rarely used clinically because of difficulty obtaining informed consent from acutely manic patients.
- Also highly effective for bipolar depression.
- No controlled data available, but some data show efficacy as maintenance treatment for treatment-resistant bipolar patients.
- Details on its techniques and side effects are described in Chapter 3 (pp. 55–56, 68–69).

Combination Treatments

- Bipolar disorder is treated with polypharmacy more often than any other psychiatric disorder.
- Combinations are used often for acute mania, bipolar depression, and maintenance treatment.
- For acute mania, controlled data demonstrate that a combination of lithium or valproate plus an antipsychotic agent is significantly more effective than lithium or valproate alone.
- For maintenance treatment, preliminary evidence demonstrates that lithium plus valproate is more effective than lithium alone.
- Preliminary evidence suggests that a combination of lithium or valproate plus olanzapine is more effective than lithium or valproate alone in preventing manias.

- For acute mania, commonly prescribed combinations are:
  - √ Lithium plus antipsychotic.
  - √ Valproate plus antipsychotic.
  - √ Lithium plus antiepileptic drug.
  - √ Lithium plus gabapentin (despite lack of evidence for efficacy).
  - √ Valproate plus gabapentin.
  - √ Two antiepileptic drugs (e.g., valproate plus carbamazepine).
  - √ Lithium or antiepileptic drug plus high-potency benzodiazepine (e.g., clonazepam).
- For bipolar depression, commonly prescribed combinations are:
  - √ Two mood stabilizers.
  - √ Any mood stabilizer plus antidepressant.
    - □ Most common combination treatment.
- For maintenance treatment, commonly prescribed combinations are:
  - √ Lithium plus valproate.
  - √ Lamotrigine plus any other antiepileptic drug or lithium
    - □ The assumption is that lamotrigine is more effective in preventing depressions, and the other mood stabilizers are more effective in preventing manias.
  - √ Lithium or antiepileptic drug plus atypical antipsychotic.
  - √ Any mood stabilizer plus gabapentin.

PHASES OF TREATMENT

Acute

- First-line agents for treating acute manic or hypomanic episodes:
  - √ Lithium.
  - √ Valproate.
  - √ Atypical antipsychotics, especially olanzapine.
- Response rates over a 3-week period: 40–60%.
- To diminish symptoms of mania as quickly as possible, prescribe a combination of lithium or valproate plus an antipsychotic (most commonly, olanzapine or risperidone).
- High-potency benzodiazepines (especially clonazepam) or gabapentin can be prescribed adjunctively to decrease activity and help ensure sleep.
  - √ These should not be considered primary antimanic agents.

- Hypomania
  √ Can be treated less aggressively, with slower dose titration.
  √ Clonazepam and gabapentin can be prescribed, as with mania.
- Compliance can be a major problem in treating acute mania/hypomania (given the common euphoria and lack of insight).
- Electroconvulsive therapy (ECT):
  √ Effective for acute mania.
  √ Rarely used because of patients' reluctance to consent to treatment.

Continuation

- Purpose: to prevent relapse soon after clinical improvement.
- No studies have examined optimum continuation treatment.
- Consensus is 6–12 months as reasonable continuation therapy following a manic or hypomanic episode.
- Many patients need maintenance treatment.

Maintenance

- Purpose: long-term prevention of manias and depressions.
- Necessary for virtually all patients following even a single manic episode.
  √ Future risk of relapse is > 85%.
- Possible exceptions are patients with:
  √ Medication-induced mania (e.g., from antidepressants, stimulants, steroids).
  √ Hypomanic rather than manic episode.
- Therapeutic plan is typically based on a combination of efficacy data, clinician preference, patient preference, and side-effect profile.
- Lithium, valproate:
  √ Most well-documented efficacy.
  √ Use as first-line agents.
- Carbamazepine, olanzapine, oxcarbazepine:
  √ Some evidence of efficacy as maintenance treatment.
  √ Use as second-line maintenance treatments.
- Lamotrigine may have selective efficacy in preventing depressions.
  √ For bipolar patients who are depression prone (i.e., depressions are worse or far more frequent than manias), consider lamotrigine.

BIPOLAR DISORDER

- Combination therapies:
  - √ Helpful for patients who have repeated breakthrough manias.
  - √ Use either two mood stabilizers or combination of mood stabilizer plus adjunctive antipsychotic.
- Breakthrough episodes in maintenance treatment:
  - √ Very common.
  - √ Evaluate the efficacy of maintenance treatment not just by elimination of any subsequent mood episodes, but by indications of:
    - □ Fewer episodes.
    - □ Milder episodes.
    - □ More interepisode stability.

Compliance

- √ Major problem, largely due to lack of insight into illness and side effects of medications.
- √ To enhance compliance, attempt to involve patients as much as possible in treatment planning.
- √ Keep in mind that female patients are particularly unlikely to comply with medications that produce substantial weight gain.

TREATMENT CONSIDERATIONS FOR WOMEN OF REPRODUCTIVE-AGE

- Obtain initial menstrual history:
  - √ Typical cycle length.
  - √ Typical duration of menses.
- Instruct patient to chart menstrual cycles after initiating treatment (e.g., with chart such as in Figure 7.1), especially after initiating valproate or prolactin-elevating antipsychotic medications.
- Monitor patient's symptoms in relation to menstrual cycle.
  - √ If patient experiences recurrent premenstrual relapse or exacerbation of bipolar disorder, obtain serum medication levels during follicular phase (i.e., 10–14 days after onset of menses) and again in the premenstrual phase.
  - √ If the premenstrual level is lower than follicular level, consider increasing medication dose at midcycle.
- Heterosexual women who take mood stabilizers and are sexually active:
  - √ If recent unprotected sex, obtain immediate pregnancy test.

- ▫ OTC pregnancy tests are 99% accurate at 12–14 days post conception.
- ✓ Educate about risks of medication exposure to fetus if patient becomes pregnant.
- ✓ Encourage patient to use contraception regularly if she does not wish to conceive.
- Consider obtaining assessments of weight in medication management visits.
  - ✓ Medication-induced weight gain may lead to noncompliance with treatment.
  - ✓ Weight gain is associated with adverse health consequences, including hypertension, hyperlipidemia, and diabetes.
  - ✓ Obesity in women who conceive is linked with an increased risk of neural tube defects in the newborns.
  - ✓ BMI (body mass index): weight in kg divided by height in meters, squared):
    - ▫ BMI of 25–29.9: overweight.
    - ▫ BMI of 30 or more: obese.

Drug Interactions

- Interactions between antiepileptic drugs (AEDs) and reproductive hormones:
  - ✓ Medications that induce hepatic enzymes produce greater clearance of oral contraceptives (OCs) and hormonal contraception (HRT) and can thus reduce their efficacy (see Table 4.2).

Table 4.2. Interactions between Antiepileptic Drugs, Oral Contraceptives (OC), and Hormone Replacement Therapy (HRT)

AEDs Prescribed for Bipolar Disorder That Induce Metabolism of OC or HRT:

carbamazepine
oxcarbazepine
topiramate

AEDs Prescribed for Bipolar Disorder That Do Not Induce Metabolism of OC or HRT:

valproate
gabapentin
lamotrigine

- Women with bipolar disorder who take these AEDs should be advised:
  - ✓ If using birth control pill, use a high-dose formulation (i.e., 50 mcg/day of estradiol).
  - ✓ If receiving medroxyprogesterone injections (Depo-Provera), obtain injection every 10 weeks rather than every 12 weeks.
  - ✓ Consider addition of a barrier form of contraception (e.g., condom, diaphragm).
- Midcycle spotting while on the birth control pill may signify ovulation; a barrier method for contraception should be added if this occurs.
- Postmenopausal women taking these AEDs (Table 4.2) may need higher doses of hormone replacement to reduce vasomotor symptoms (e.g., hot flashes, night sweats).
- Oral contraceptives can reduce lamotrigine levels by 40–60% (through the effect of estrogen on glucuronide-conjugating enzymes).
  - ✓ Women on oral contraceptives may therefore require higher doses of lamotrigine.
  - ✓ If they discontinue the oral contraceptive, they may require a subsequent adjustment of the lamotrigine dosage.

TREATMENT OF BIPOLAR DISORDER DURING PREGNANCY

- No mood stabilizer currently has FDA approval for use during pregnancy.
- FDA use-in-pregnancy categories for medications are listed in Table 1.4.
- FDA use-in-pregnancy ratings for mood stabilizers are listed in Table 4.3; FDA use-in-pregnancy ratings for additional medications (e.g., benzodiazepines, antidepressants) are listed in Table1.5.
- The decision to use a mood stabilizer during pregnancy ultimately depends on:
  - ✓ The risks of bipolar disorder on the mother and fetus.
  - ✓ Research findings on the safety/risks of medication use in pregnancy.
- Perform and record a careful risk–benefit discussion (see Table 1.3).
- Women with long periods of stability between mood episodes may be able to taper and discontinue mood stabilizers prior to

Table 4.3. Food & Drug Administration Use-in-Pregnancy Ratings for Mood Stabilizers

Medication	FDA Use-in-Pregnancy Rating
lithium (Lithobid, Eskalith, lithium carbonate)	D
valproate (Depakote, Depakene)	D
carbamazepine (Tegretol)	D
gabapentin (Neurontin)	C
lamotrigine (Lamictal)	C
oxcarbazepine (Trileptal)	C
olanzapine (Zyprexa)	C

conception and remain medication-free during most, if not all, of the pregnancy.

- Ideally, medications should be tapered over at least 4 weeks to avoid the risk of relapse associated with abrupt medication discontinuation.

- Patients who decide to taper and discontinue medications during pregnancy should be clearly informed about the risk of relapse. Ultimately, the patient makes the decisions about the course of treatment and the risks she is willing to face during the pregnancy.

- Educate patients about ways to maximize chances of conception by using methods to detect ovulation (e.g., monitoring basal body temperature or using an OTC ovulation detection kit).

- Women with severe bipolar disorder who face an unacceptable risk of relapse if the medication is discontinued may need to remain on medication throughout pregnancy.

- Consider electroconvulsive therapy (ECT) as an alternative to medication during pregnancy (see pp. 55–56).

- Recommend folic acid (folate) supplementation (minimum 0.6 mg/day) for all women who are trying to conceive; women on valproate and carbamazepine should take much higher dose: 4 mg/day.

- Prescribe medications in divided doses during pregnancy (rather than single daily doses) to avoid peak serum concentrations.

- Antipsychotic medications are an alternative to mood stabilizers for treating bipolar disorder during pregnancy (see pp. 85–86).

- To report exposures to antiepileptic drugs during pregnancy and obtain the latest information available, call the Antiepileptic Drug Pregnancy Registry at 888-233-2334; for exposures to lamotrigine, also call Glaxo SmithKline at 800-722-9292.

- Make use of all available nonpharmacological interventions (e.g., psychotherapy, couples therapy, bipolar support groups), as they may reduce the likelihood of relapse during pregnancy.

BIPOLAR DISORDER

Lithium Use in Pregnancy

- First-trimester use of lithium is associated with approximately a 1–7% risk of miscellaneous cardiovascular malformations, including:
  - √ Ebstein's anomaly: defect in the formation of the tricuspid valve of the heart.
    - ▫ Generally occurs in approximately 1 in 20,000 live births, but the rate increases up to 20-fold in infants exposed to lithium in first trimester.
  - √ Coarctation of aorta.
  - √ Left–right ventricular disproportion.
  - √ Ventricular septal defect.
  - √ Cardiomegaly.
  - √ Patent ductus arteriosus.
  - √ Mitral atresia.
- The following have been reported for some newborns exposed to lithium during pregnancy (but the exact risk is unknown):
  - √ Preterm birth.
  - √ Macrosomia.
  - √ Neonatal hypotonia and lethargy.
  - √ Neonatal hypoglycemia.
  - √ Neonatal cyanosis.
  - √ Polyhydramnios.
  - √ Thyroid depression and goiter.
  - √ Diabetes insipidus.
  - √ Bradycardia.
  - √ Electrocardiogram abnormalities.
- Effects are usually transient, lasting 1–2 weeks (reflecting the serum half-life of lithium in newborns, which is approximately 5–6 times longer than in adults).
- If lithium is used in first trimester, obtain a fetal echocardiogram and high-resolution ultrasound between gestational weeks 16–18.
- Prescribe lithium in multiple daily doses (preferably using a sustained-release preparation) to avoid exposing fetus to peak blood levels.
- Follow serum lithium levels at least monthly.
  - √ Changes in glomerular filtration rate and fluid volume in pregnancy can lead to a reduction of serum lithium levels as pregnancy progresses.
  - √ Adjust medication dose accordingly.

- The mother's lithium dose may need to be reduced in the 1–2 weeks prior to estimated date of delivery to avoid maternal lithium toxicity following the rapid fluid loss and reduction in lithium clearance that occur with delivery.
- A study of 5-year-old children exposed to lithium during pregnancy reported no evidence of developmental abnormalities.

Valproate and Carbamazepine Use in Pregnancy

- Use in the first 6 weeks is linked with approximately a 2–3% risk of neural tube defects (NTDs).
  √ A 10–20-fold increase compared to general prevalence of NTD.
- Risk remains after controlling for increased risk of congenital malformations due to epilepsy.
- Valproate-induced NTDs are usually severe open spinal defects, such as sacral or lumbosacral spina bifida, and are often complicated by other defects in the central nervous system (e.g., hydrocephaly).
- Women of reproductive age who take these medications should be strongly advised to use reliable methods of contraception.
- Whenever possible, avoid use of valproate or carbamazepine during pregnancy or postpone their use until after the 6th gestational week, at which time neural tube closure is completed.
- The teratogenic potential of these drugs appears to result, at least in part, from their antifolate activity and free radical metabolites (e.g., arene oxide, epoxide metabolites).
- Other potential risks to infant associated with prenatal use of valproate and carbamazepine:
  √ Developmental delay.
    □ Lower scores on cognitive testing, greater need for additional educational services.
    □ Particularly documented for valproate.
  √ Craniofacial defects.
    □ Midface hypoplasia, high forehead, short nose, low-set ears.
  √ Cardiovascular defects.
  √ Fingernail hypoplasia.
  √ Hypospadia.
  √ Hepatic dysfunction.
- "Fetal valproate syndrome" refers to cardiovascular, craniofacial, urogenital, digital, respiratory tract anomalies and developmental

delays that have been observed in children born to epileptic women who took valproate during pregnancy.

- If valproate or carbamazepine must be used during the first 6 weeks of pregnancy:
  - √ Inform patient of the risks of congenital malformations associated with the use of these medications in pregnancy.
  - √ Keep the doses as low as possible.
  - √ Prescribe medication in divided doses to avoid high peak levels.
  - √ Patient should take folic acid supplementation 4 mg/day (i.e., 5–10x the usual recommended dose).
    - □ Begin this supplementation prior to conception and continue at least through week 12 of gestation.
  - √ Between 16–18 weeks gestation, obtain the following diagnostic tests:
    - □ Alpha-fetoprotein and acetylcholinesterase analysis from amniotic fluid (rather than from serum, which is less sensitive); levels are typically elevated if a neural tube defect is present.
    - □ Anatomic ultrasound.
  - √ These combined diagnostic techniques typically detect 92–95% of neural tube defects.
- Monitor valproate and carbamazepine levels at least monthly.
  - √ Changes in protein binding, hepatic metabolism, and fluid volume in pregnancy can lead to a reduction of serum levels as pregnancy progresses.
  - √ Adjust medication dose accordingly.
- Valproate and carbamazepine also can produce a deficiency in vitamin K-dependent clotting factors (II, VII, IX, X), with subsequent increased risk of bleeding disorders in the fetus and newborn.
  - √ The mortality rate of postnatal bleeding is high because it is typically not noticed until the infant is in shock.
  - √ Prescribe vitamin K (10–20 mg/day) to the mother during the last trimester of pregnancy.
  - √ At birth, the newborn should receive a 1 mg injection of vitamin K.
  - √ If newborn's vitamin K-dependent factors are under 25% of normal values, intravenous administration of fresh frozen plasma may be necessary.

Use of Newer Antiepileptic Drugs in Pregnancy: Gabapentin, Lamotrigine, Oxcarbazepine, Topiramate

- Little human data available.
- Most information on prenatal exposures is for lamotrigine: No adverse effects have been observed in the infants.
- Lamotrigine has antifolate effects in animal studies but apparently not in humans.
- Other new AEDs do not appear to produce antifolate effects but data on this question are limited.
- Except for tiagabine, these new AEDs do not produce free radical metabolites.
- However, more human data are necessary before these medications can be considered safe to use in pregnancy.

Use of Atypical Antipsychotic Agents in Pregnancy

Some data exist for olanzapine use in pregnancy (see p. 151).

Alternative Treatments for Bipolar Disorder in Pregnancy

- Verapamil (Calan, Isoptin):
  - ✓ Reported to be effective for mania in some studies.
  - ✓ Relative to other mood stabilizers, its mood-stabilizing effect is probably weak.
  - ✓ Verapamil is used to treat hypertension during pregnancy and to inhibit preterm labor (by decreasing uterine contractility).
  - ✓ From available data, verapamil does not appear to be teratogenic and may be an alternative to traditional mood stabilizers during pregnancy.
- Omega-3 fatty acids:
  - ✓ Polyunsaturated fatty acids found in plants and fish, particularly cold-water, oily fish (e.g., salmon, tuna, halibut); also present in nuts and green leafy vegetables.
  - ✓ Include: eicosapentaenoic acid (EPA) and docosahexanoic acid (DHA).
  - ✓ Unlike monounsaturated fats, omega-3 fatty acids present numerous health benefits, including improvement of cardiovascular health and reduced risk of preterm birth.

BIPOLAR DISORDER

Table 4.4. Child Homicide in the United States

Neonaticide	Killing of newborn on the day of birth; related more to social than psychiatric factors (e.g., young naive women who have concealed the pregnancy)
Homicides during 1st week of life	Usually by mother
Homicides occurring after 1st week of life	Usually by father or stepfather
Homicides of toddlers/older children	Usually by someone unrelated to child

Source: (Overpeck MD, Brenner RA, Trumble AC, Trifiletti LB, Berendes HW. Risk factors for infant homicide in the United States. *N Engl J Med.* 1998;339:1211–1216.)

√ An adequate supply of maternal omega-3 fatty acids is necessary to support optimal neurological development of fetus.

  □ When supplied in infant formula at adequate doses, they appear to improve infant cognitive development and visual acuity.

√ Have been helpful as adjunctive treatment of bipolar mania in one study.

√ May provide a safe adjunctive treatment for bipolar disorder during pregnancy and breast-feeding.

TREATMENT OF BIPOLAR DISORDER FOLLOWING DELIVERY

- Risk for relapse of bipolar I disorder (mania or depression) is 30–70% in first 4–6 weeks postpartum.
- Risk of postpartum relapse of bipolar spectrum disorders (e.g., bipolar II disorder) has not been established.
- Bipolar prophylaxis should begin in third trimester of pregnancy or immediately after delivery (if the patient is not already on a mood stabilizer).
- Because sleep deprivation may precipitate a relapse of illness, nighttime awakenings should be kept to a minimum.
  √ Ideally, another household member (e.g., the partner/spouse; a live-in nanny) should help with infant's nighttime feedings (e.g., with pumped breast milk or formula).
- The University of Rochester's Lactation Study Center (585-275-0088) maintains a database that provides information to physicians regarding medication use and potential risks during breast-feeding.

Postpartum Psychosis

- Rare; incidence 0.1–0.2% of all births.
- Serious illness requiring immediate hospitalization!

- Risks:
  - √ History of bipolar or schizoaffective disorder (principal risk factor).
  - √ First birth.
- Symptomatology:
  - √ Delusions (e.g., that the child is dead or was exchanged for another child).
  - √ Paranoia.
  - √ Catatonic excitement.
  - √ Sleep disturbance.
  - √ Confusion.
  - √ Mood lability.
  - √ Restlessness.
  - √ Hallucinations (including command hallucinations to do something to the child).
- Risk of infanticide estimated at 4%.
- Generally better outcome than psychotic disorders occurring at other times in a woman's life, particularly if onset is within 3 weeks of delivery.
- Approximately 37–50% of cases follow a multiphasic course (i.e., three or more subsequent episodes).
- Most common long-term course in these cases is schizoaffective or bipolar disorder.
- Need for long-term treatment is controversial in women with no previous psychiatric illness.

Treatment of Pospartum Psychosis
- Mood stabilizers.
- Antipsychotic agents.
- Antidepressants (if delusional depression).

BIPOLAR DISORDER

USE OF MOOD STABILIZERS DURING BREAST-FEEDING

Lithium

- Generally contraindicated during breast-feeding.
- Breast milk levels have reached 24–72% of mother's serum levels.
- Cyanosis, hypotonia, EKG changes have been reported in nursing infants exposed to lithium through breast-feeding.
- Lithium can reach toxic serum levels in the nursing infant during periods of fluid loss (e.g., diarrhea, vomiting, fever).
- Infants' immature kidney function limits lithium excretion.

- Some clinicians use lithium in breast-feeding women with very close follow-up of the infant's serum levels and monitoring for dehydration and signs of lithium toxicity.

Valproate

- On basis of limited data, valproate appears generally safe to use during breast-feeding.
- Thrombocytopenia and hepatotoxicity have been reported in three infants exposed to valproate through breast milk.
- It is advisable, but not absolutely necessary, to monitor liver function tests and complete blood count in nursing infants exposed to valproate.

Carbamazepine

- On basis of limited data, carbamazepine appears generally safe to use during breast-feeding.
- Case reports have described drowsiness and poor sucking in nursing infants exposed to carbamazepine.
- One report described hepatitis in an infant exposed to carbamazepine through breast milk.
- It is advisable, but not absolutely necessary, to monitor liver function tests in nursing infants exposed to carbamazepine.

Lamotrigine

- Excreted in considerable amounts in breast milk.
- Infant serum levels approximately 30% of maternal levels.
- Best not to use in breast-feeding women, particularly given the risk of life-threatening rashes (risk is higher in children than in adults).

New Antiepileptic drugs

- Little is known about safety of gabapentin, topiramate, and other new AEDS in breast-feeding.
- Best not to use these agents in breast-feeding women.

Antipsychotic Agents

- Some data exist for olanzapine and haloperidol in breast-feeding (see Chapter 6).
- Almost no data exist for risperidone, ziprasidone, quetiapine, and clozapine in breast-feeding.

General Principles for Use of Mood Stabilizers During Breast-Feeding

- Choose medications for which safety data exist on their use in breast-feeding.
- Prescribe the minimum dosage of medication that produces remission of mother's symptoms.
- Consider supplementation with bottle-feeding to reduce infant's exposure.

Factors That Influence Infant's Exposure to Medication Through Breast Milk

- Maternal dose:
  - √ Medications should be maintained at the lowest effective dose to minimize the infant's exposure.
- Timing of maternal dose:
  - √ Concentrations of some drugs are known to peak a few hours after maternal ingestion of the medication; however, the time when medications peak in breast milk is unknown for most medications used for bipolar disorder.
- Medication properties:
  - √ Half-life (see Table 4.5).
    - □ Shorter half-life typically produces less exposure.
  - √ Protein binding (see Table 4.5).
    - □ Higher protein binding typically produces less exposure.

Nursing Infant Serum Concentrations of Medication

- Infant serum concentrations provide a measure of infant's exposure.
- However, the blood draw can be traumatic to the infant, and the information is of limited value, as no cutoff has been established for a safe serum level of medication in infants.

Table 4.5. Pharmacokinetic Parameters of Medications Used for Bipolar Disorder

Medication	Protein Binding (%)	Half-Life (hrs)*
lithium	N/A	12–27
valproate	> 90	4–17
carbamazepine	75	11–24
gabapentin	0	5
lamotrigine	50	29
olanzapine	93	21–54
oxcarbazepine	40	8–11
topiramate	13–17	21

* With monotherapy; half-life can vary with drug interactions.

- Therefore, these serum levels need not be obtained routinely in a nursing infant.
- However, the data may provide reassurance for some mothers, especially if the concentration is very low or undetectable.
- To obtain an infant serum concentration of medication:
  √ Wait until medication serum levels are likely to be at steady state (i.e., at least five medication half-lives).
  √ Ask the laboratory to use a high-sensitivity assay (i.e., with a limit of detection < 2 ng/ml).
  √ Measure concentrations of both the parent drug and its metabolites in infant serum.

TREATMENT CONSIDERATIONS FOR PERI- AND POSTMENOPAUSAL WOMEN

- Mood stabilizers may exacerbate risk of osteoporosis/osteomalacia:
  √ Valproate and carbamazepine are linked with a reduction of bone-mineral density and increased risk of bone fractures (see pp. 75, 83).
  √ Lithium may (theoretically) increase the risk for osteoporosis because of risk of hyperparathyroidism and subsequent loss of bone calcification.
    □ In the absence of hyperparathyroidism, lithium does not pose such risk.
- Medications that induce hepatic enzymes (see Table 4.2) produce greater clearance of hormone replacement therapy (HRT) and can thus reduce its efficacy.
  √ Postmenopausal women who take these medications may need higher doses of hormones to reduce hypoestrogenemia-induced vasomotor symptoms (e.g., hot flashes, night sweats).

TREATMENT CONSIDERATIONS FOR ELDERLY WOMEN

- See Chapter 1, pages 18–19.
- Optimal plasma level for geriatric patients:
  √ Acute treatment: 0.4–0.8 mEq/l.
  √ Maintenance treatment: 0.3–0.8 mEq/l.
- Elderly women may respond to blood levels of lithium that would be considered subtherapeutic for younger patients (e.g., 0.4 mEq/l).

- Lithium levels and clinical signs of toxicity should be monitored closely in elderly women.
  √ Toxicity can occur at lower blood levels compared to younger adults.
- Carbamazepine and oxcarbazepine-induced hyponatremia occurs more frequently in elderly patients.

BIPOLAR DEPRESSION

- An important consideration in the treatment of bipolar depression is the potential risk that antidepressants may precipitate mania/hypomania or accelerated cycling and mood destabilization in bipolar patients.
- Greater risks of antidepressant-induced mania from tricyclics vs. the newer antidepressants.
- Adding an antidepressant to a mood stabilizer confers far less risk for switching compared to antidepressant alone for bipolar I patients.

Options for Bipolar Depression

- Mood stabilizers:
  √ Lamotrigine has best data as acute antidepressant.
  √ Lithium.
    □ Demonstrated efficacy in early studies (1960s–1970s); results from recent studies have been inconsistent.
    □ Delayed time to efficacy (up to 8 weeks).
    □ More popular in Europe than in United States as acute antidepressant.
  √ Valproate, carbamazepine, oxcarbazepine, gabapentin, topiramate: all with inconclusive data.
- Antidepressants:
  √ General paucity of controlled studies examining risks/benefits of antidepressants in bipolar disorder.
  √ Overall efficacy likely to be similar to that seen with unipolar depression.
  √ SSRIs.
    □ Evidence of efficacy.
    □ Evidence of relatively low switch rates (< 10%) when added to mood stabilizers.
    □ Fluoxetine's long half-life makes it impossible to discontinue quickly if patient switches into mania.

BIPOLAR DISORDER

    ✓ Venlafaxine.
        ▫ Preliminary evidence of efficacy.
        ▫ Evidence of low switch rate in bipolar II depression.
    ✓ Bupropion.
        ▫ Evidence of efficacy and relatively low switch rate.
    ✓ Tricyclics.
        ▫ Conflicting evidence of efficacy.
        ▫ Evidence of highest switch rate among antidepressant classes.
    ✓ MAOIs.
        ▫ Evidence of efficacy.
        ▫ Switch rate may be as high as tricyclics, but switches appear to be milder.
- Electroconvulsive therapy (see Chapter 3, pp. 55–56).

5. Anxiety Disorders and Insomnia

INTRODUCTION

Anxiety disorders are the most common psychiatric conditions in the United States. Approximately one in 10 people suffer from them, with the rate in women two to three times that of men. Several reasons have been suggested for the preponderance of anxiety disorders in women, including the conflicting demands of work and family, differential treatment of self-sufficiency and assertiveness in girls compared with boys, histories of physical and sexual abuse, the impact of shifting levels of reproductive hormones, and under-reporting of anxiety by men. Progesterone metabolites (e.g., allopregnanolone) are potent enhancers of GABA in the central nervous system and produce anxiolytic and hypnotic effects. As their levels drop (e.g., premenstrually, postpartum) women may experience heightened vulnerability for anxiety. Exposure to traumatic experiences (e.g., assault, injury to self or loved one) also contributes to the increased prevalence of anxiety disorders in women. Although the lifetime exposure to traumatic events is slightly higher in men, women face twice the likelihood of developing posttraumatic stress disorder.

Pharmacotherapy plays a dominant role in the treatment of some anxiety disorders. In this chapter, we address panic disorder, generalized anxiety disorder, social anxiety disorder, obsessive–compulsive disorder, and posttraumatic stress disorder—those disorders for which the evidence for pharmacological efficacy is strong. Specific phobias are not covered because there is no evidence that medications play a significant role in their treatment.

In evaluating women with anxiety disorders, it is important to screen for the use of medications and other substances that may produce anxiety, such as appetite suppressants, decongestants, antihypertensive agents, corticosteroids, herbal supplements, and caffeine-containing beverages. Certain medical conditions that predominate in women, such as thyroid disorders and systemic lupus erythematosus, may also produce anxiety.

The clinical course of many anxiety disorders differs among men and women. Posttraumatic stress disorder (PTSD) is more likely to be chronic in women, whereas obsessive–compulsive disorder (OCD) is more likely to be chronic in men. Women with panic disorder experience more recurrences of the illness and are more likely to develop agoraphobia. Comorbid psychiatric disorders also generally differ by gender: Comorbid depression is more common in women with anxiety disorders, whereas comorbid substance and alcohol use disorders are more common in men. Comorbid psychiatric disorders are particularly likely with generalized anxiety disorder (GAD) and PTSD.

Maternal anxiety during pregnancy has been linked with a heightened risk for preterm labor and low birth weight, even after controlling for variables such as socioeconomic status, maternal weight gain, and health habits during pregnancy. Corticotropin releasing hormone (CRH), which rises during stress, is centrally involved in the initiation of parturition. Pregnant women who experience high levels of stress and the concomitant elevated levels of stress hormones may experience a premature initiation of labor. Additionally, elevated stress hormones increase susceptibility to intrauterine vaginal infections, which in turn are associated with premature rupture of membranes and preterm labor.

Little is known about the course of anxiety disorders during pregnancy or following delivery. Available data show that panic disorder follows a variable course in pregnancy but usually worsens in the postpartum period. Symptoms of OCD typically worsen during pregnancy and following delivery. Little data exist about the course of GAD, PTSD, or specific phobias during pregnancy and the postpartum period.

Postpartum anxiety disorders can be accompanied by severe insomnia and restlessness and may be confused with postpartum psychosis.

Women with severe postpartum anxiety may endorse fears—usually involving the newborn—that seem excessive and unrealistic, adding to the possibility of a misdiagnosis of postpartum psychosis.

Despite the universal role of anxiety in all the anxiety disorders, the relationship among these disorders has been difficult to delineate. Partly, this difficulty reflects the recency of our diagnostic system of anxiety disorders. Panic disorder, for example, did not become a formal diagnosis until 1980. The frequent comorbidity between the anxiety and depressive disorders has led some observers to attempt to create unifying schemes, as was common in the past. With comorbidity rates of 60–85%, primarily with other anxiety and mood disorders, GAD is the prototype disorder that seems to overlap with others. Genetic/family studies indicate some specificity for the disorders but not with complete consistency, thereby supporting both the "lumpers" and the "splitters" for anxiety diagnoses. British psychiatry particularly has been critical of the current splitting of anxiety disorders in the *DSM-IV*. Adding to this issue are the increasing data showing equal efficacy of antidepressant medications for both depression and most of the anxiety disorders.

Recommendations regarding long-term treatment of the different anxiety disorders are far more tentative than those for mood disorders or schizophrenia because of the relative paucity of studies in this area. Nonetheless, evidence for the chronic or recurrent nature of anxiety disorders is emerging, as is the need for long-term treatment. Many of the medications used to treat anxiety disorders are classified as antidepressants. They are listed in this chapter with specific prescribing instructions. Side effects are covered in other chapters and are so noted.

PHARMACOLOGICAL TREATMENT OF ANXIETY DISORDERS

Panic Disorder

- The goals of pharmacotherapy are to decrease or eliminate panic attacks, anticipatory anxiety, phobic avoidance, and depression.
- Relapse of panic attacks is relatively common (averaging 50%) even among patients maintained on long-term treatment.
- Associated agoraphobia, when present, is likely to be chronic and is best treated with cognitive–behavioral therapy.

Table 5.1. Pharmacotherapy for Panic Disorder

Medication Class	Advantages	Disadvantages
SSRIs	Excellent documentation of efficacy High patient acceptance Once daily dosage	Delayed onset of action Stimulant side effects
Benzodiazepines	Early onset of action (especially for anticipatory anxiety) Well-tolerated High patient acceptance	Sedation Cognitive side effects Withdrawal difficulties
Tricyclic antidepressants	Clinical experience for decades Once daily dosage	Delayed onset of action Substantial side effects Stimulant side effects with some agents
MAOI	Antiphobic effects?	Dietary and medication restrictions Substantial side effects

- Table 5.1 shows the three classes of effective treatments, each with specific advantages and disadvantages.
- After improvement in symptoms, consensus recommendation (based mostly on clinical experience rather than research data) is for 12–18 months of continuation treatment.
- Consider maintenance (i.e., indefinite) treatment for:
  √ Patients with chronic symptoms.
  √ Patients who have a past history of relapse after medication discontinuation.
- If medications are discontinued, taper slowly over 1–2 months to reduce likelihood of relapse or withdrawal symptoms (except for fluoxetine, which does not need to be tapered gradually because of its long half-life).

SSRIs

- Dominant treatment for panic disorder because of patient acceptance, ability to treat comorbid depression (if present), good tolerability, lack of dependency, and lack of withdrawal problems with most agents.
- Double-blind placebo-controlled studies show efficacy for citalopram, fluoxetine, fluvoxamine, paroxetine, sertraline. Preliminary data also show efficacy with S-citalopram.
- Although efficacy across SSRIs appears to be similar, consider using less stimulating medications (e.g., paroxetine, citalopram).
- If patient is desperate for immediate relief, consider initiating treatment with tranquilizer (e.g., benzodiazepine or gabapentin)

along with SSRI for immediate benefit and to combat SSRI-induced stimulation.
√ Discontinue the tranquilizer after SSRI takes effect.
- Dosing:
  √ Patients with panic disorder are more sensitive to side effects than depressed patients, especially to SSRI-induced stimulation.
  √ Therefore, start with lower doses than for depression—e.g., half or even one-quarter of usual antidepressant starting dose (see p. 37).
  √ Full antipanic doses are similar to antidepressant doses, but some patients appear to respond to very low doses (e.g., paroxetine or citalopram 5 mg/day).
- Potential side effects: see page 39.

Benzodiazepines

- Well-established efficacy for panic disorder.
  √ Additionally beneficial for reduction of anticipatory anxiety.
- Often used in combination with antidepressants for panic disorder.
- Most data are for alprazolam; studies using clonazepam, lorazepam, and diazepam are also positive, indicating probable class effect.
- May be effective for depression that develops subsequent to panic disorder.
- Potential for dependence and withdrawal are a concern for many clinicians (see section below on GAD).
- Patients with panic disorder do not appear to require escalating doses of benzodiazepines over time.
- Dosing: See Table 5.3 and section below on GAD.
- Potential side effects: See section below on GAD.

Tricyclics

- Oldest treatment for panic disorder.
- Well-established efficacy in many controlled trials for decreasing (or eliminating) panic attacks and reducing anticipatory anxiety and phobic avoidance.
- Delayed onset (typically at least 4–6 weeks)
- All tricyclics are likely to be effective, but most data are for imipramine.

- Dosing:
  - √ Start with low dose (e.g., imipramine 10 mg/day).
  - √ Increase more slowly for panic disorder than for depression, due to panic patients' increased sensitivity to side effects.
  - √ Effective doses vary but appear to be somewhat lower than doses used for depression.
    - ◻ E.g., typical doses of imipramine for panic disorder are 50–200 mg/day (vs. 100–300 mg/day for depression).
- Potential side effects: See page 42.

MAOIs

- Rarely used for panic disorder.
- Some studies from pre-*DSM-III* era indicate probable efficacy, but no conclusive data.
- Unclear effective dose range, compared to antidepressant doses.
- Side-effect profile and dietary restrictions sorely limit patient acceptance.

Other Medications

- Preliminary data suggest efficacy for valproate and gabapentin, with doses adjusted according to clinical response and side effects.

Generalized Anxiety Disorder (GAD)

Table 5.2 describes three first-line pharmacotherapeutic options for GAD and several second-line options.

- Response typically occurs in 3–6 weeks, sometimes sooner.
- Benzodiazepines typically produce slightly earlier responses than buspirone, SSRIs, or venlafaxine.
- Consider long-term (i.e., indefinite) treatment, as GAD tends to be chronic.

Table 5.2. Pharmacotherapy for Generalized Anxiety Disorder

First-Line Agents	Second-Line Agents
Benzodiazepines	Gabapentin
Buspirone	Tricyclic antidepressants
Serotonergic antidepressants	Atypical antipsychotics
(SSRIs, venlafaxine)	Antihistamines (e.g., diphenydramine)
	Nonbarbiturate tranquilizers
	Barbiturates

Table 5.3. Benzodiazepine Doses

Generic Name	Trade Name	Usual Dosage Range (mg/day)
alprazolam	Xanax	0.5–4
chlordiazepoxide	Librium	10–100
clonazepam	Klonopin	0.5–3
clorazepate	Tranxene	7.5–60
diazepam	Valium	5–40
estazolam	ProSom	1–2
flurazepam	Dalmane	15–30
halazepam	Paxipam	40–160
lorazepam	Ativan	1–6
oxazepam	Serax	15–90
quazepam	Doral	7.5–15
temazepam	Restoril	15–30
triazolam	Halcion	0.125–0.5

✓ Patients typically experience a waxing/waning course with remission between episodes, or chronic mild symptoms with periods of exacerbation.

Benzodiazepines

Short-term efficacy appears equivalent for all agents in the class. Table 5.3 lists the benzodiazepines and their usual doses.

• More effective for somatic symptoms (e.g., trembling, sweating, tension, insomnia) than psychological symptoms (e.g., worry, apprehension) of anxiety.

• Differ from each other in speed of onset of action, elimination half-life, and method of metabolism (see Table 5.4).

• Lorazepam, oxazepam, and temazepam are rapidly metabolized (glucuronidated) and do not have active metabolites.
  ✓ Safer in patients with liver disease and nursing mothers (see p. 125).

Table 5.4. Characteristics of Benzodiazepines

Generic Name (Trade Name)	Rapidity of Effect	Half-Life
alprazolam (Xanax)	Intermediate	Intermediate
chlordiazepoxide (Librium)	Intermediate	Long
clonazepam (Klonopin)	Intermediate	Intermediate–long
clorazepate (Tranxene)	Rapid	Long
diazepam (Valium)	Rapid	Long
estazolam (ProSom)	Rapid	Intermediate
flurazepam (Dalmane)	Intermediate	Long
halazepam (Paxipam)	Slow	Long
lorazepam (Ativan)	Intermediate	Intermediate
oxazepam (Serax)	Intermediate–slow	Intermediate
quazepam (Doral)	Rapid	Long
temazepam (Restoril)	Intermediate	Intermediate
triazolam (Halcion)	Intermediate	Short

Dosing

- Start with low dose and gradually increase, as needed and tolerated.
- After patients reach effective dosage range, symptoms improve quickly (i.e., within 1–3 days).
- Dosage regimen (once daily vs. multiple doses) depends on medication's half-life:
  - √ Administer short half-life agents bid–qid.
  - √ Long half-life agents can be prescribed once daily.
- For chronic treatment, use doses that are same or slightly lower than for acute (i.e., initial) treatment.

Potential Side Effects

- Sedation:
  - √ Tolerance to sedation typically develops over first few weeks.
- Cognitive impairment.
- Psychomotor incoordination:
  - √ Associated with an increased rate of motor vehicle accidents, falls in elderly.
  - √ Side effects are additive with those of alcohol, causing potential for higher risk of motor vehicle accidents, falls.
- Depression:
  - √ Rare; seen occasionally at high doses.
- Disinhibition/rage:
  - √ More common in elderly, children, and brain-damaged individuals.

Dependency/Withdrawal Effects

- Clinicians and patients are often concerned about the "addictive" nature of benzodiazepines.
- However, tolerance to benzodiazepines' anxiolytic effects (i.e., requirement for higher doses over time) is unusual.
- Abuse of benzodiazepines is also unusual:
  - √ Except among patients with prior histories of sedative/hypnotic abuse or alcohol abuse/dependence.
- Physical dependence and withdrawal symptoms (if the medication is stopped abruptly) are relatively common.
- Predictors of withdrawal difficulties are listed in Table 5.5.
- Withdrawal symptoms:
  - √ Tremulousness.
  - √ Anxiety.
  - √ Rarely, seizures (especially if a short-acting benzodiazepine is stopped suddenly after prolonged use).

Table 5.5. Factors Predicting Benzodiazepine Withdrawal Symptoms

Medication Predictors	Patient Predictors
Longer time on drug	Current anxiety and depressive symptoms before medication discontinuation
Short half-life	Dependent personality traits
Abrupt withdrawal (vs. taper)	History of alcohol or drug (especially sedative) abuse
High dose	Past experience with benzodiazepines

- Time course of withdrawal is dependent on half-life of agents:
  - √ Short half-life agents are associated with withdrawal symptoms within 24 hours of first missed dose.
  - √ Longer half-life agents produce withdrawal symptoms after 2–3 days of lowered dose or discontinuation.

Strategies to Avoid Benzodiazepine Withdrawal Symptoms
- Taper slowly (up to many months with some patients).
- Switch to equivalent amount (see Table 5.6) of longer half-life benzodiazepine (if patient is on short half-life agent) and then taper.
- Add carbamazepine 200–600 mg/day or valproate 500–1000 mg/day, then taper.
- Initiate adjunctive cognitive–behavior therapy.

Buspirone

- Anxiolytic with mechanism of action through serotonergic receptors.
- Unrelated to benzodiazepines; therefore, does not block benzodiazepine withdrawal.
- Many older studies demonstrated efficacy in treating generalized anxiety; recent studies indicate less efficacy.

Table 5.6. Equivalent Doses Among Benzodiazepines

Generic Name	Dose (mg)
alprazolam	0.5
chlordiazepoxide	10–15
clonazepam	0.25–0.5
diazepam	5
lorazepam	1
oxazepam	15
temazepam	15

- May be more effective against psychological symptoms than physical symptoms of anxiety (in contrast to benzodiazepines).
- Delayed onset of action (a few weeks—in marked contrast to benzodiazepines); patients should be educated to expect a delayed effect.
- In many clinicians' experience, buspirone is less effective than other antianxiety agents.
- Prior exposure to benzodiazepines may predict poorer response to buspirone.
- Remarkably well tolerated.
- No interaction with alcohol.
- No cognitive impairment or psychomotor incoordination.
- No withdrawal effects; can be discontinued without tapering.
- No dependence or potential for abuse.

Dosing
- Start at 5 mg tid or 10 mg bid.
- Increase by 5–10 mg weekly.
- Aim for usual dose of 30–60 mg/day, usually prescribed twice daily.

Potential Side Effects
- Dizziness (typically, a few hours after each dose).
- Headache.
- Nausea.

SSRIs and SNRIs

- Solid evidence of efficacy (and FDA indication) for paroxetine and venlafaxine.
- Likely that all other serotonergic antidepressants are also effective.
- However, fluoxetine and sertraline may produce excessive stimulation in first few days of treatment.
- Time to onset of efficacy: usually 2–4 weeks.
- Doses for GAD are similar to antidepressant doses (see p. 37).
- Side effects: See pages 38–39.

Gabapentin

- Virtually no studies have examined its use for GAD. Nevertheless, it is increasingly prescribed both on prn and daily dosing schedule.

- Dosing: Optimal dose range for GAD is unclear, but is usually prescribed at 300–2400 mg/day, occasionally as high as 3600 mg/day.
- Side effects: See p. 87.

Tricyclic Antidepressants

- Clear evidence of efficacy but rarely used because of side effects and lack of promotion by pharmaceutical companies.
- Delayed time to onset, typically 4–6 weeks.
- Dosing: Use somewhat lower doses than for depression (see p. 37).
- Side effects: See page 42.

Antihistamines

- Diphenhydramine (Benadryl) and hydroxyzine (Atarax, Vistaril) are the most commonly prescribed.
- Infrequently used for anxiety.
- Useful primarily for patients for whom benzodiazepines should not be prescribed (e.g., history of alcohol abuse).

Dosing
- Diphenhydramine and hydroxyzine: 25 mg bid, titrate up to 50 mg qid.

Potential Side Effects
- Sedation.
- Blurry vision.
- Dry mouth.
- Dizziness.

Antipsychotics

- Essentially no studies, but increasingly used for GAD.
- Typically reserved for severe, treatment-resistant anxiety.
- Virtually all use of antipsychotics for anxiety involves atypical agents: risperidone, olanzapine, and quetiapine.
- Dosing: Usually much lower than usual antipsychotic doses (e.g., use 10–25% of usual doses; see pp 134–140).
- Side effects: See pages 135–140.

Social Anxiety Disorder (SAD)

- Treatment approaches differ depending on whether patient has generalized vs. limited form of the disorder.

- Most data (and most of this section) addresses generalized SAD—i.e., a generalized fear of social or performance situations.
- Limited form is discussed in the following section.
- Onset of efficacy occurs over 3–6 weeks.
- Consider long-term (indefinite) treatment, as many patients relapse after discontinuation of short-term pharmacotherapy.

SSRIs

- Most commonly prescribed trcatment for social anxiety disorder.
- Efficacy best-documented for paroxetine (which has FDA indication for social anxiety disorder), but all SSRIs are likely to be effective.
- Dosing: Similar to treatment for depression; see pages 37–38.
- Side effects: See p. 39.

MAOIs

- Phenelzine has best documentation, but all MAOIs appear to be similarly effective.
- Dosing: Similar to treatment for depression; see page 43.
- Use is limited by dietary restrictions, side effects; see pages 44–45 for details.
- Reversible MAOIs ("RIMAs," reversible inhibitors of MAO-A, unavailable in United States) appear effective, but less so than irreversible MAOIs such as phenelzine.

Benzodiazepines

- Efficacy best demonstrated for clonazepam.
- Weaker evidence for alprazolam.
- Dosing: moderate to high doses (e.g., 4 mg/day of clonazepam or alprazolam).
- Use is limited by concerns about physical dependence, sedation, withdrawal problems.

Gabapentin

- Efficacy demonstrated in one study, using high doses (3600 mg/day).
- Typically used as second-line agent.
- See pages 86–87 for details.

Other Medications

- Venlafaxine and bupropion may be effective.
- Use doses similar to antidepressant doses (see p. 37).

Limited Social Anxiety Disorder

- Essentially, pertains to stage fright/performance anxiety.
- Effectively treated with prn use of beta-blockers.

Beta-Blockers

- Propranolol is most commonly used.
- Atenolol is occasionally used.
- Instruct patient to take medication approximately 1 hour prior to performance.
- Try test dose before actual event.
- Contraindicated in patients with asthma or congestive heart failure.

Dosing
- Propranolol 10–80 mg/day.
- Atenolol 50–100 mg/day.

Potential Side Effects
- Sedation.
- Hypotension.
- Slow heartbeat.
- Shortness of breath, wheezing.
- Cold hands and feet.
- Depression.

Obsessive–Compulsive Disorder

- All currently effective first-line pharmacotherapies strongly increase CNS serotonin.
- Response rate approximately 60%.
- *Response* typically defined as 25–35% improvement on symptom rating scale.
- Remission is rare, therefore the appropriate endpoint (i.e., when has maximum benefit been achieved?) is difficult to ascertain.
- Therapeutic effects require longer treatment than for depression or other anxiety disorders.
- May take up to 12 weeks for maximal response.

- Prescribe medications at doses approximately 2–3 times higher than for treating depression.
- Consider maintenance treatment, as OCD is typically chronic, with waxing/waning intensity and high relapse rate when successful pharmacotherapy is discontinued.

SSRIs

- Most commonly prescribed class of medications for OCD.
- Well-documented efficacy for fluoxetine, fluvoxamine, sertraline, paroxetine.
  √ Citalopram is probably also effective.
- All agents are probably equally effective.

Dosing
- Increase over a few weeks to relatively high daily doses:
  √ Citalopram 40–60 mg/day.
  √ Fluoxetine 40–60 mg/day.
  √ Fluvoxamine 200–250 mg/day.
  √ Paroxetine 40–60 mg/day.
  √ Sertraline 150–200 mg/day.
- If inadequate response after 6 weeks, increase to higher doses:
  √ Citalopram 80 mg/day.
  √ Fluoxetine 80 mg/day.
  √ Fluvoxamine 300 mg/day.
  √ Paroxetine 60–80 mg/day.
  √ Sertraline 200–250 mg/day.

Potential Side Effects
- See pages 39–40.
- OCD patients tolerate medications more easily than depressed patients.

Clomipramine

- Only tricyclic that is effective for OCD, secondary to strong serotonergic effect.
- At least equal efficacy to SSRIs.
- Usually prescribed second line due to side effects.

Dosing
- Start 25–50 mg hs.
  √ Increase by 25–50 mg increments over 7–14 days, as tolerated, to 150 mg/day.

- If inadequate response after 6 weeks, increase by 50 mg increments every few weeks to 250 mg/day.

Potential Side Effects
- See pages 39 and 46 for details.
- Caution re: increased risk of seizures at high dose (> 250 mg/day).

Other Treatments

- Clear evidence for efficacy of cognitive–behavioral therapy with specific technique of exposure and response prevention.
- Weak support for MAOIs.
- Preliminary evidence for venlafaxine.

Strategies for Treatment-Resistant OCD
- Multiple strategies have been explored but few validated.
- Efficacy of second SSRI after failure of the first is not well-studied, but appears to be occasionally effective.
- If SSRI (or two SSRIs) is ineffective, try clomipramine, and vice versa.
- Best-validated adjunctive approach: Add an antipsychotic to either SSRI or clomipramine.
  - √ Either risperidone or olanzapine appear effective in low doses (1–4 mg/day or 2.5–10 mg/day, respectively) for OCD, regardless of presence of comorbid tics or psychosis.
  - √ Conventional antipsychotics (e.g., haloperidol) are effective adjuncts for OCD with comorbid tics.
- Combine SSRI plus clomipramine.
  - √ Caution re: potential effect of SSRI in raising clomipramine blood levels.
    - □ Monitor clomipramine levels.
- Initiate cognitive–behavioral therapy.
- Augmentation strategies with either weak or negative findings in studies include lithium, buspirone, trazodone, and clonazepam.

Posttraumatic Stress Disorder (PTSD)

SSRIs

- Best-documented, most commonly prescribed treatments.
- Sertraline and paroxetine have FDA indication for PTSD.
- Fluoxetine also effective in controlled studies.
- All SSRIs likely to be equivalently effective.

ANXIETY DISORDERS AND INSOMNIA

- Positive effects seen gradually over 4–8 weeks.
- Efficacy seen for numbing/avoidance as well as reexperiencing/intrusion and hyperarousal.
- Dosing: Use doses similar to treatment for depression (see p. 37).

Antianxiety Agents

- Benzodiazepines are often prescribed adjunctively to decrease arousal, insomnia.
- However, studies show no evidence of efficacy for other symptoms of PTSD.
- Caution re: benzodiazepine withdrawal effects (particularly with short-acting agents, such as alprazolam), as they can exacerbate symptoms of PTSD.
- Consider using longer-acting benzodiazepines (see Table 5.4).

Other Agents

- Positive (but relatively weak) effects for amitriptyline.
- MAOIs are somewhat effective, but not for numbing/avoidance, and are generally prescribed third-line because of dietary restrictions, drug restrictions, and side-effect profile.
- Lamotrigine (average dose 380 mg/day) was effective in a small, controlled study.
- Open trials show efficacy for carbamazepine, valproate, and lithium.
- Antipsychotic medications have not been studied for PTSD but are sometimes prescribed for aggressive and self-destructive behaviors.

TREATMENT CONSIDERATIONS FOR WOMEN OF REPRODUCTIVE AGE

- Obtain initial menstrual history:
  - □ Typical cycle length.
  - □ Typical duration of menses.
- Monitor patient's symptoms in relation to menstrual cycle:
  - √ If patient experiences recurrent premenstrual relapse or exacerbation of anxiety, consider increasing medication dose by 50% at midcycle.

√ Blood levels of certain antidepressants have been reported to vary across the menstrual cycle.

□ If the patient reports a recurrent relapse or exacerbation of the anxiety disorder, consider measuring the concentration premenstrually and in the follicular phase of the menstrual cycle (for medications with well-established therapeutic ranges, e.g., TCAs).

□ If serum antidepressant concentration is found to drop premenstrually, consider increasing the medication dosage at midcycle.

* Monitor whether the patient's menstrual cycle changes following initiation of an antidepressant:

√ Consider instructing patients to chart menstrual cycles (e.g., with chart such as Figure 7.1 p. 159) after initiating certain medications.

√ Serotonergic antidepressants can increase prolactin levels and produce irregular menses and amenorrhea.

□ Possible exception of sertraline, because its dopaminergic effects may offset the impact on prolactin.

√ Conversely, benzodiazepines may restore normal menstrual cycling in women with stress-induced anovulation.

* Heterosexual women who take antidepressants and are sexually active:

√ If recent unprotected sex, obtain immediate pregnancy test.

√ OTC pregnancy test 99% accurate at 12–14 days postconception.

√ Educate about risks of medication exposure to fetus if patient becomes pregnant.

√ Encourage patients to use contraception regularly if they do not wish to conceive.

TREATMENT OF ANXIETY DISORDERS DURING PREGNANCY

* Review patient's likelihood of a psychiatric relapse during pregnancy and postpartum period.
* If a woman has a history of severe relapse of anxiety disorder following medication discontinuation, the medication may need to be continued throughout the pregnancy.
* Attend to factors that may underlie anxiety during pregnancy (e.g., marital conflict, work-related stresses).

- Cognitive–behavioral therapy is an effective treatment for many patients with panic disorder and OCD and should be considered as an alternative to medication.
- Additional nonpharmacological interventions include elimination of caffeine and nicotine, reduction of psychosocial stressors, and family and/or couples therapy.
- Perform and record a careful risk–benefit discussion of treatment considerations (see Table 1.3).

Use of Anxiolytic and Antidepressant Medications During Pregnancy

- No anxiolytic or antidepressant currently has FDA approval for use during pregnancy.
- FDA use-in-pregnancy categories for medications are listed in Table 1.4.
- FDA use-in-pregnancy ratings for specific psychiatric medications, including anxiolytics and antidepressants, are listed in Table 1.5.
- The decision to use an anxiolytic or antidepressant during pregnancy ultimately depends on:
  √ The risks of continued anxiety on the mother and fetus.
  √ Research findings on the safety/risks of medication use in pregnancy.

Benzodiazepines

- Conflicting reports of risk—some data have described a slightly increased risk of oral clefts when benzodiazepines are used in first trimester of pregnancy.
  √ If the risk is genuine, it appears to be small, raising the risk of oral clefts from approximately 6 in 10,000 (0.06%) to approximately 7 in 1,000 (0.7%).
  √ Reported particularly for diazepam and alprazolam.
- Use of benzodiazepines in late pregnancy has been associated with hypotonicity and respiratory depression in newborns.
- Whenever possible, attempt to minimize or avoid the use of benzodiazepines during weeks 5–10 of the pregnancy, as this is the time when the fetal lip and palate form.
- Occasional use of small doses of benzodiazepines during pregnancy does not appear to be associated with neonatal complications.

- Lorazepam is a reasonable choice in pregnancy:
  - √ No active metabolites.
  - √ Appears to cross into the placenta at a lower rate than do other benzodiazepines.
- To reduce the risk of toxicity and withdrawal symptoms in the neonate, minimize the use of benzodiazepines near term.
- To avoid in utero withdrawal, benzodiazepines should be tapered, rather than discontinued abruptly, during pregnancy.

Buspirone (Buspar)

- No human data available.

Antidepressants

- See pages 50–58.

TREATMENT OF ANXIETY DISORDERS DURING BREAST-FEEDING

Use of Anxiolytics During Breast-Feeding

Benzodiazepines

- Little data available.
- Most reports have involved clonazepam and temazepam; less frequently, alprazolam, diazepam, lorazepam.
- Most case reports have not described adverse effects in nursing infants.
- These adverse effects include decreased respiration rate, lethargy, and cyanosis.
  - √ Symptoms resolved with discontinuation of nursing.
- If benzodiazepines are used during nursing, dosage and length of use should be minimized.
- Best to use short-acting agents without active metabolites (e.g., lorazepam, oxazepam) to minimize risk of sedation in infant.

Other Anxiolytic Medications

- A case series (N = 5) reported no adverse effects in nursing infants whose mothers took zolpidem.

Antidepressants

- See pages 59–62.

TREATMENT CONSIDERATIONS FOR PERI- AND POSTMENOPAUSAL WOMEN

- Vasomotor symptoms may produce shortness of breath, increased heart rate, and disrupted sleep.
  √ May be mistaken for anxiety attacks.
- If a perimenopausal patient develops new-onset anxiety or insomnia, ask whether she is experiencing vasomotor symptoms such as hot flashes or night sweats. If so, hormone replacement therapy (HRT) (see Chapter 9) may be helpful.
- If symptoms have not remitted after 7–10 days of HRT, consider initiating usual treatment for anxiety.
- Of note, venlafaxine, paroxetine, and fluoxetine have been reported to significantly reduce hot flashes (independent of their effects on mood or anxiety).

TREATMENT CONSIDERATIONS FOR ELDERLY WOMEN

- See pages 18–19.
- Benzodiazepines, particularly those with long half-lives (see Table 5.4), should be prescribed with caution in elderly women because of the risk of:
  √ Accumulation.
  √ Daytime sedation.
  √ Cognitive decline.
  √ Psychomotor incoordination.
  √ Paradoxical disinhibition/rage.
  √ Falls.

TREATMENT OF INSOMNIA

The prevalence of chronic insomnia in women is approximately 1.3 times higher than in men. Women are more likely to experience insomnia during certain phases in their reproductive lives: for example, during the week prior to menses women may sleep poorly because of premenstrual cramping and bloating. In the third trimester of pregnancy, women often have difficulty lying comfortably as they sleep.

In perimenopausal women, night sweats can cause multiple awakenings. Additional causes of insomnia include depression and anxiety disorders and medication side effects.

- Distinguish between different etiologies of insomnia:
  - √ Primary sleep disorders (e.g., sleep apnea, restless legs syndrome).
  - √ Medical disorders (e.g., asthma, chronic obstructive pulmonary disease, sleep apnea).
  - √ Medications (e.g., bronchodilators, blood pressure medications, decongestants, corticosteorids, theophylline, beta-blockers).
  - √ Substance use/abuse.
  - √ Psychiatric disorder (40–75% of all insomnias).
  - √ Idiopathic (primary) insomnia.
  - √ Disruptions in circadian rhythm (e.g., from jet lag or rotating work shifts).
  - √ Perimenopausal hot flashes, night sweats.
  - √ Premenstrual cramping.
- If sleep problems are associated with somatic symptoms in the premenstrual phase of the menstrual cycle, a low-dose oral contraceptive or an analgesic may help.
- If sleep problems are related to night sweats, hormone replacement will help.
- Controversy as to primary goal of therapy: improved subjective sleep quality vs. improvement in sleep architecture.
- Vast majority of medications have been tested only in the short term (over a period of a few weeks).
  - √ Ongoing use of hypnotics for months or years is very common.
- Encourage sleep hygiene (i.e., healthy sleep habits):
  - √ Eliminate caffeine and nicotine.
  - √ Maintain same bedtime and wake-up times.
  - √ Avoid napping in the day.
  - √ Maintain regular exercise.
  - √ Avoid excessive fluids in the evening.
  - √ Go to bed only when sleepy.
  - √ Use bed only for sleep and sex.
  - √ Increase exposure to natural/bright light during day.
  - √ Make sure bedroom is quiet and comfortable.
  - √ Do not go to bed hungry or full.

- Try behavioral sleep therapies.
  - √ E.g., sleep restriction therapy (behavioral technique to increase sleep efficiency).
- For insomnia due to a sleep disorder (e.g., sleep apnea) or medical or psychiatric disorder, treat the primary disorder.
- Medications discussed below are typically prescribed for primary insomnia or in association with psychiatric disorders when adjunctive sleep aid is needed.
- Many psychiatric patients complain of insomnia, even after the psychiatric disorder has been treated.

Pharmacological Options for Insomnia

- Benzodiazepines.
- Selective benzodiazepine agonists.
- Sedating antidepressants.
- Sedating antihistamines.
- Atypical antipsychotics.
- Natural compounds.

Benzodiazepines

- Although only four agents—estazolam, lorazepam, temazepam, and triazolam—are marketed as hypnotics, all agents in the class are equally effective
- See Table 5.3 for list of benzodiazepines and their doses.
- Individual agents differ in speed of onset of action and half-life; see Table 5.4.
- Prescribe shorter half-life agents for insomnia uncomplicated by daytime anxiety.
- Use caution (especially in elderly) with long half-life benzodiazepines because of risk of accumulation, daytime sedation, cognitive decline, and falls.
- Taper when discontinuing after prolonged use.
  - √ Rebound insomnia is common following sudden discontinuation after prolonged use.

Selective Benzodiazepine Agonists

- Zolpidem (Ambien) and zaleplon (Sonata).
- Active only at GABA-A/benzodiazepine type I receptors (benzodiazepines are active at both receptors) and probably have less

anxiolytic, anticonvulsant, and muscle-relaxing effects than benzodiazepines.
- Both are very short half-life agents.
  √ Zolpidem's half-life: 2–3 hours.
  √ Zaleplon's half-life: 1–2 hours (shortest of all hypnotics).
- Short half-life (especially of zaleplon) allows potential middle of night use without significant morning sedation/hangover.

Antidepressants

- Marked increase in clinical use of antidepressants as hypnotics over the last 15 years, despite paucity of studies.
- Mechanism of efficacy may involve both antidepressant/ antianxiety effects as well as sedating side effects.
- Trazodone is most commonly used at low doses: 25–200 mg/day.
- May be combined with other antidepressants.

Antihistamines

- Diphenhydramine (Benadryl) and hydroxyzine (Atarax) are the most commonly prescribed.
- Relatively rapid tolerance to hypnotic effect occurs in most patients; these medications are usually not very helpful over extended time periods.
- Dosing: See page 117.
- Side effects: See page 117.

Antipsychotics

- No systematic studies available.
- Consider low doses of sedating atypical antipsychotics (e.g., olanzapine 2.5–5 mg hs; quetiapine 100–200 mg hs) for intractable insomnia.

Natural Compounds

- Melatonin:
  √ Data inconsistent regarding its hypnotic efficacy.
- Valerian root:
  √ Only mildly sedating and hypnotic.

6. Schizophrenia

Gender differences are well-documented in the clinical presentation and course of schizophrenia. In general, women with schizophrenia show better premorbid functioning and experience a more benign course of illness and a higher quality of life. They are more likely than men to marry and to obtain education and employment. The average age of onset of the illness is older in women, peaking at ages 25–35, compared to 18–25 years in men. Gender differences in the prevalence of schizophrenia remain inconclusive. Some studies have reported a greater prevalence of the illness in men, particularly when the population has consisted primarily of young adults. When older individuals are included in epidemiological surveys, the male excess appears to be balanced out by the greater prevalence of late-onset schizophrenia in women.

Several researchers have hypothesized that estrogen reduces women's vulnerability to the illness. In support of this hypothesis is the observation that late-onset schizophrenia (i.e., beyond age 45, a time when estrogen levels are declining) occurs predominantly in women. Furthermore, levels of estrogen have been found to inversely correlate with greater symptomatology, and estrogen supplementation has been reported to improve the illness. Estrogen supplementation appears effective in potentiating the response to antipsychotic medications among pre- and postmenopausal women, and may also reduce the symptoms of tardive dyskinesia.

Significant gender differences also arise in the pharmacological treatment of schizophrenia. Antipsychotic medications produce certain side effects that are unique to, or more common in, women, including menstrual irregularities and galactorrhea. Treatment response may vary across the menstrual cycle, requiring adjustments such as premenstrual increases in medication dosage. In general, women respond more favorably to treatment than men.

The expression of symptoms also appears to vary by gender. Compared to men, women are more likely to experience positive symptoms and less likely to experience negative symptoms. Positive symptoms refer to experiences that do not reflect reality, such as delusions and hallucinations, whereas negative symptoms include deficits in feelings (affective flattening), initiative/interest (avolition), and thinking/verbal expressiveness (alogia and impoverished thought content). Additional dimensions of psychopathology in schizophrenia include clinically significant depressive symptoms—which occur more commonly in women—and cognitive deficits, e.g., in verbal processing, which are more common in men. These differences in symptom expression probably explain, at least in part, women's better social functioning and response to treatment.

Women with schizophrenia are frequently unaware of the appropriate use of contraception and are at risk for unintended pregnancies. Maternal schizophrenia is linked with an increased risk for poor perinatal outcome (e.g., low birth weight; preterm delivery and stillbirth) that is not fully explained by factors such as health behaviors, access to care, maternal age, parity, and education. Compared to the general population, women with schizophrenia face a higher likelihood of giving birth to children with neural tube defects—possibly because of inadequate dietary folate intake and obesity, two risk factors for neural tube defects that are prevalent among chronically mentally ill women. Psychotic denial of pregnancy may occur, particularly in women with previous histories of loss of children to foster care or adoption. Some reports describe an improvement of symptoms during pregnancy, possibly as a result of increased visits with health-care professionals, but little prospective information is available on the course of the illness in pregnant women.

Antipsychotic medications were among the first of our modern psychopharmacological agents. First explored as treatments for psychotic agitation, they were quickly discovered to decrease the positive symptoms of schizophrenia. Unfortunately, soon thereafter, the medications' relative lack of efficacy for negative symptoms and their considerable side-effect burdens became equally clear. Nonetl antipsychotics became the mainstay of treatment for schizophre the 1990s, the emergence of the second generation of antipsychɔ ̠ ̠ ̠— the so-called "atypical" agents—shifted the risk–benefit ratio for treatment. These new agents are at least as effective as the older agents and are generally better tolerated. They are less likely to elevate prolactin and therefore present safer choices for the long-term treatment of female patients. Nonetheless, there is still an enormous need for safer and more effective treatments for schizophrenia.

Antipsychotics are frequently used in the treatment of psychotic disorders other than schizophrenia (e.g., psychotic mania). Increasingly, the newer antipsychotics are also used to treat nonpsychotic syndromes, including bipolar disorder, borderline personality disorder, severe anxiety and insomnia, and as adjunctive treatment for depression. Compared to the older agents, the new antipsychotics' lower side-effect burden—rather than greater efficacy—has led to their increasing acceptance in the treatment of nonpsychotic disorders.

ANTIPSYCHOTIC AGENTS

Classification

- Typical (or conventional, i.e., older agents) vs. atypical agents.
- Definition of atypicality remains ambiguous but generally refers to agents which, compared to conventional agents, have:
  - √ Fewer extrapyramidal symptoms.
  - √ More serotonin-blocking effects.
  - √ Less reliance on pure dopamine-2 blockade.
  - √ Fewer secondary negative symptoms, such as depression or akinesia.
- Atypical agents differ from each other structurally and biologically and should each be placed in a separate category, but they share clinical traits, including efficacy and side-effect profiles.
- Conventional agents may be classified by chemical structure— e.g., phenothiazines, butyrophenones—but these classifications are clinically meaningless.
- They are more logically grouped by potency—i.e., the number of milligrams needed for a clinical response.

SCHIZOPHRENIA

Table 6.1. Antipsychotic Doses

Generic Name (Trade Name)	Starting Dose (mg)	Dose Range (mg)
Atypical Agents		
aripiprazole (Abilify)	15	15–30
clozapine (Clozaril)	25	200–600
olanzapine (Zyprexa)	5–10	10–25
quetiapine (Seroquel)	50	400–800
risperidone (Risperdal)	1–2	2–8
ziprasidone (Geodon)	20–40	120–160
Conventional Agents: Low Potency		
chlorpromazine (Thorazine)	25–50	300–600
mesoridazine (Serentil)	25	150–300
thioridazine (Mellaril)	25–50	300–600
Conventional Agents: Middle Potency		
loxapine (Loxitane)	10–25	40–200
molindone (Moban)	10–25	40–200
perphenazine (Trilafon)	4–8	16–48
thiothixene (Navane)	2–5	10–50
trifluoperazine (Stelazine)	2–5	10–50
Conventional Agents: High Potency		
fluphenazine (Prolixin)	1–5	2–15
haloperidol (Haldol)	1–5	2–15
Long-Acting Injectable Agents		
fluphenazine decanoate (every 2 weeks)	6.25	6.25–25
haloperidol decanoate (every 4 weeks)	50	50–200

Table 6.2 compares antipsychotic side effects across different antipsychotic medications.

Factors to Consider in Choosing an Antipsychotic

- Atypical agents should be chosen as first-line for the majority of patients:
  - √ Only exception: Patient with excellent prior response to conventional agents or who does well specifically with long-acting injectable conventional agent.
  - √ All atypical antipsychotics are equivalently effective.
    - □ Except for clozapine, which is most effective.
  - √ However, individual patients may respond better to one antipsychotic than another.
- Side-effect profile:
  - √ May be used therapeutically; e.g., prescribe a sedating antipsychotic for an anxious/agitated patient.

Table 6.2. Side-Effect Ratings of Antipsychotic Medications

Generic Name (Trade Name)	Extrapyramidal Symptoms (EPS)	Sedation	Anticholinergic Effects	Postural Hypotension	Weight Gain
Atypical Agents					
risperidone (Risperdal)	+	+	+	+	+
olanzapine (Zyprexa)	0–+	+++	+	+	+++
quetiapine (Seroquel)	0	++	+	+	+
ziprasidone (Geodon)	0–+	+	0–+	0–+	0
aripiprazole (Abilify)	0	+	0–+	0–+	0
clozapine (Clozaril)	0	+++	++	++	+++
Conventional Agents: Low Potency					
Class includes: chlorpromazine (Thorazine) mesoridazine (Serentil) thioridazine (Mellaril)	+	+++	+++	++	+++
Conventional Agents: Middle Potency					
Class includes: loxapine (Loxitane) molindone (Moban) perphenazine (Trilafon) thiothixene (Navane) trifluoperazine (Stelazine)	++	+–++	++	++	++
Conventional Agents: High Potency					
Class includes: fluphenazine (Prolixin) haloperidol (Haldol)	+++	+	+	+	+

0 None; + Minimal; ++ Moderate; +++ Significant

- Individual and family history of response.
- Medical considerations.
- Safety in overdose.
- Cost:
    √ Depends on patient's financial means, insurance coverage, potential formulary issues (via insurance).

- For women of reproductive age, plans regarding pregnancy:
  √ If patient plans to conceive in near future, try to use medications with safety data for use during pregnancy.
- Comorbid psychiatric conditions.
- Potential for drug interactions.

Risperidone (Risperdal)

- First atypical agent, released in 1994.
- In addition to tablets, is available in a liquid formulation.

Dosing
- Average dose 4–4.5 mg/day.
- In acute psychosis, start risperidone 1 mg bid.
- Increase by 1 mg every 2–3 days, as needed and tolerated.
- Recent study suggests 2 mg/day is as effective as 4 mg/day, with fewer side effects.
- Length of full trial is 8 weeks:
  √ Partial response occurs within 1–2 weeks.
- Once acute episode ends, consider switching to evening dosing for maintenance treatment.

Potential Side Effects
- Hyperprolactinemia (see pp. 143–45)
- Extrapyramidal symptoms (EPS; see p. 145 for details):
  √ Produces the highest rate of EPS among atypical agents.
  √ Dose related; rate of EPS increases significantly above 6 mg/day.
- Sedation.
- Weight gain.
- Nasal stuffiness.
- Tardive dyskinesia: (p. 145)
  √ Infrequent.
  √ Risk is significantly less than for typical antipsychotics.
  √ Unknown relative risk compared to other atypical agents.

Olanzapine (Zyprexa)

- Commonly used for many psychiatric disorders.
- Among atypical agents, has best documentation of efficacy for nonschizophrenic disorders, e.g., bipolar disorder.
- Women may respond better than men to olanzapine, possibly because of greater prevalence of affective symptoms in women.

- In addition to standard tablets, is available as an orally disintegrating tablet (Zydis).

Dosing
- For acute psychotic states, start with 5 mg bid or tid if agitation is prominent.
  √ Otherwise, start with 5 mg in evening and increase, as tolerated, up to 10–20 mg/day.
- Average dose is 14–17 mg/day.
- For maintenance treatment, start with 5 mg daily and increase by 5 mg increments to 10–15 mg daily dose.
  √ For most patients, high doses (> 25 mg/day) do not appear to be more effective than usual doses.

Potential Side Effects
- Sedation:
  √ Prescribe olanzapine at bedtime, unless daytime sedation/tranquilization is required (e.g., for psychotic agitation or mania).
- Weight gain:
  √ May be very problematic.
  √ Maximal in first 6 months, then levels off.
  √ Average weight gain: 10 lbs in 10 weeks.
  √ Those with lower weight pretreatment are at higher risk to gain more weight.
- New-onset type II diabetes mellitus and hyperlipidemia:
  √ Found in most studies.
  √ Usually associated with medication-induced weight gain.
  √ Monitor fasting blood glucose and lipid panel (see Table 6.3).
  √ Frequency of monitoring not yet established; monitoring should be based on:

Table 6.3. Laboratory Monitoring of Patients on Olanzapine

Fasting Plasma Glucose Levels for Nonpregnant Women:
Normal < 110 mg/dl
Impaired fasting glucose 110 and 125
Diabetes if > 125

Fasting Lipid Levels (Ideals):
Total cholesterol: < 200 mg/dl
HDL cholesterol: > 60 mg/dl
LDL cholesterol: < 130 mg/dl
Triglycerides: < 200 mg/dl

Table 6.4. Risk Factors for Diabetes

Family history
Obesity
Hypertension
Previous gestational diabetes or delivery of a baby over 9 lb
Ethnic group: African American, Hispanic, Native American,
  Pacific Islander, and Asian American at greater risk than
  Caucasian

- □ Risk factors for diabetes (see Table 6.4).
- □ Signs/symptoms suggesting hyperglycemia or diabetes (see Table 6.5).
- Elevation of serum prolactin:
  √ Generally minimal.
- Extrapyramidal side effects:
  √ Risk is minimal except at very high dose (> 25 mg/day).
- Tardive dyskinesia:
  √ Risk is very low.

Quetiapine (Seroquel)

- Prescribed less frequently than risperidone or olanzapine because fewer studies have examined its use.
- Initial concern about potential cataract development (seen in beagle dogs exposed to quetiapine) has not been borne out by clinical experience—no evidence of increased risk in humans.

Dosing

- Package insert instruction for initial dose is probably too low for acutely psychotic inpatients.
- Start 50 mg bid and increase, as tolerated (optimally over 1 week), to 400–600 mg/day.
- If insufficient response after 2 weeks, consider increasing to 600–800 mg/day.

Potential Side Effects

- Sedation (more than risperidone, less than olanzapine).
- Mild orthostatic hypotension.

Table 6.5. Signs and Symptoms of Diabetes

Frequent urination
Excessive thirst
Tingling or numbness in hands and feet
Slow-healing bruises
Recurring infections (e.g., skin, bladder, gum)

- Weight gain.
- Hyperprolactinemia (minimal).
- Very low to no extrapyramidal symptoms.

Ziprasidone (Geodon)

- Released in 2001; less overall experience than with agents listed above.

Dosing
- Start with 20 mg bid; increase by 20 mg every 1–2 days to 120–160 mg/day.
- Concern among clinicians about less efficacy compared to other antipsychotics may be due to inadequate dosing (60–80 mg/day instead of 120–160 mg).
- Ongoing studies are exploring the use of higher doses (up to 320 mg/day).
- Short-acting intramuscular preparation was released in late 2002 for use in emergency rooms and inpatient settings for immediate tranquilization.

Potential Side Effects
- Stimulation:
  - √ Similar to anxiety, possibly represents akathisia.
  - √ May explain the sense of lesser efficacy, if patient and/or doctor expect the sedation/tranquilization that occurs with other antipsychotics.
- Increased corrected QT (QTc) interval:
  - √ Ziprasidone is associated with greater QT prolongation than other atypical antipsychotics, but this risk is relatively small.
  - √ Increased QTc interval can lead to risk of potentially fatal cardiac arrhythmia (Torsade de pointes).
  - √ Pretreatment EKG not required, but some clinicians and patients request it.
  - √ Do not use ziprasidone with other QT-prolonging drugs.
  - √ Probably wise to avoid in patients at risk for electrolyte disturbances (e.g., those with active eating disorder), because they may be at increased risk of QT prolongation and arrhythmia.
  - √ Probably wise to avoid ziprasidone as first-line agent in patients with
    - ▫ Cardiac conduction defects.
    - ▫ History of recent myocardial infarction.

- Family history of unexplained sudden death (may be genetic long QT interval).
- No extrapyramidal symptoms.
- No weight gain—this is an important advantage compared to other agents.
- Risk of tardive dyskinesia unknown; theoretically, should be very low.

Aripiprazole (Abilify)

- Released in early 2003; limited experience so far.
- Unique mechanism of action:
  - √ Partial dopamine agonist, i.e., has characteristics of both dopamine blockers and dopamine agonists.
  - √ It is unclear whether partial agonism confers superior antipsychotic effects.
  - √ This property, however, does appear to produce a lower likelihood of hyperprolactinemia, compared to other antipsychotic agents.

Dosing
- Effective range for treating psychotic disorders: 10–30 mg/day.
- Dose titration is simple: Starting dose is frequently the final dose.
- Higher doses (20–30 mg/day) are generally not more effective than lower doses (15 mg/day) for treating psychosis.

Potential Side Effects
- Nausea.
- Mild sedation.
- Stimulation effects, manifesting as anxiety, insomnia, possibly akathisia.
- Minimal weight gain.
- Minimal orthostatic hypotension.
- No extrapyramidal symptoms.
- No significant change in QTc interval.
- Minimal to no change in prolactin levels:
  - √ Appears to be the antipsychotic agent with lowest likelihood of producing hyperprolactinemia
  - √ May therefore be preferable to other antipsychotic agents for women with hormone sensitive tumors, e.g., breast cancer.

Clozapine (Clozaril)

- Most effective of all antipsychotic agents in treatment-resistant patients.
- Should never be used as first-line due to risk of life-threatening agranulocytosis.
- Efficacy against negative symptoms is most well-documented among atypical antipsychotics, but effects are still modest.
- Also appears to be the most effective agent for preventing relapses.
  - √ Unclear whether this reflects true enhanced preventive efficacy vs. better compliance secondary to lesser side-effect burden.
- Weekly or biweekly venipuncture required.
  - √ Use generally limited to committed, treatment-adherent patients.
- Among antipsychotics, has best documentation of lowering suicide rate.
- Compared to men, women taking clozapine:
  - √ Appear to reach higher blood levels, even after correction for dose and body weight.
    - □ This is particularly of concern because high concentrations of clozapine can produce seizures.
  - √ Appear to respond less well.
    - □ This may be the result of women's lower prevalence of negative symptoms, compared to men.
  - √ Appear to be at greater risk for agranulocytosis.

Dosing
- Slow: start 12.5–25 mg once daily or bid; increase by 25 mg every 2–4 days, as tolerated.
- Can switch to evening dosing, if needed to decrease daytime sedation effect.
- Typical doses are 200–500 mg/day; higher doses may be necessary for some patients.
- Clozapine plasma level > 350 ng/ml correlates with greater improvement.
- Efficacy typically occurs within 8–12 weeks, but improvement may continue over 6 months.

Potential Side Effects
- Sedation.
- Weight gain.

- Sialorrhea (hypersalivation), especially at night.
- Orthostatic hypotension.
- Constipation.
- Fever.
- Tachycardia:
  √ Responds to beta-blocker (e.g., propanolol).
- Agranulocytosis is rare but most serious side effect.
  √ Current incidence 0.38%.
  √ Fatality for agranulocytosis approximately 3%.
    □ Clozapinc is associated with fatal agranulocytosis in 1/10,000 patients.
    □ Weekly venipuncture and monitoring of blood counts are required for first 6 months of treatment.
    □ Venipuncture may subsequently be decreased to every other week.
- Seizures:
  √ Rare.
  √ Dose related, with seizure rate of 4–6% at doses > 600 mg/day.
- Cardiomyopathy:
  √ Described in case reports; incidence unknown.

Conventional Antipsychotics

- Used less frequently since the advent of atypical agents because of their greater side effect burden.
- Compared with atypical agents, they are associated with more depressive symptoms and secondary negative symptoms.
- Parenteral (injectable) haloperidol used frequently in emergency rooms and acute inpatient units.
- Two long-acting injectable preparations are currently available: fluphenazine decanoate and haloperidol decanoate.
  √ Used with outpatients who are poorly compliant with oral agents but are willing to take injections every 2–4 weeks.
  √ Should be avoided in patients at risk for pregnancy (i.e., sexually active women who do not use regular contraception).
    □ May lead to prolonged fetal exposure if the patient becomes pregnant.
- Women who are switched from conventional agents to most atypical agents may have greater chance of conception because of lowering of prolactin levels with subsequent resumption of menstrual cycling.

Dosing
- See Table 6.1.
- May increase from initial dose to full dose over days to a few weeks.
- May be prescribed once daily.
- Prescribe bid if daytime tranquilization needed.
- Parenteral haloperidol typically prescribed at 2–5 mg q 4–8 hours, as needed.
- Parenteral benztropine usually administered concomitantly to prevent dystonias, acute extrapyramidal symptoms.

Potential Side Effects
- Sedation.
- Anticholinergic effects (dry mouth, blurry vision, constipation, urinary hesitation).
- Weight gain:
  - ✓ Lower-potency agents are associated with more weight gain than high-potency agents.
- Orthostatic hypotension.
- Sexual dysfunction (e.g., anorgasmia, diminished libido).
- Hyperprolactinemia (see below).
- Amenorrhea (from prolactin elevation).
- Extrapyramidal symptoms (see p. 145).
- Tardive dyskinesia (see pp. 145–147).

Hyperprolactinemia

- Conventional antipsychotic medications can produce substantial elevation in prolactin levels through blockade of dopamine D-2 receptors in pituitary.
- Most atypical antipsychotic medications minimally change prolactin levels, with exception of risperidone.
- Women are more likely to experience antipsychotic-induced hyperprolactinemia than men.
- Antipsychotic-induced hyperprolactinemia occurs at a lower daily dose of antipsychotics in women compared to men.
- Prolactin inhibits release of FSH (see Chapter 9); therefore, hyperprolactinemia can produce menstrual cycle irregularities.
- Normal prolactin levels in women of reproductive age: 5–25 ng/ml.
- Hyperprolactinemia should be diagnosed on the basis of two separate serum prolactin levels.

Table 6.6. Differential Diagnosis of Elevated Prolactin Level

Pregnancy and nursing
Hypothyroidism
Prolactin-producing pituitary tumor (prolactinoma)
Medications, including:
 • Certain antipsychotic medications (see text)
 • Tricyclic antidepressants
 • SSRIs
 • Opiates
 • Verapamil
 • Antiemetics (e.g., metoclopramide, domperidone)
 • Hormonal contraception
Stress
Weight loss
Epilepsy
Chronic renal failure
Cirrhosis

- Prolactin levels can rise to 10 times their normal levels with use of certain antipsychotic medications.
- Elevated prolactin can result from several etiologies other than antipsychotic medications (see Table 6.6).
- Amenorrhea may occur when prolactin levels exceed 60 ng/ml.
- Galactorrhea (nipple discharge) may also occur with elevated prolactin.
- If prolactin level exceeds 100 ng/ml, consider obtaining a brain-imaging study (e.g., magnetic resonance imaging [MRI] with gadolinium enhancement) of the hypothalamic–pituitary area to rule out a prolactin-producing pituitary tumor (prolactinoma).
  √ Prolactin levels > 250 ng/ml are almost always caused by a prolactinoma.
  √ Any patient who has hyperprolactinemia, without an identified cause, should also undergo a brain-imaging study.
- Prolactin-elevating antipsychotic medications may confer a small but significant risk of breast cancer. Therefore medications producing substantial elevations of prolactin levels are best avoided in women with a history of breast cancer.

Approaches to Antipsychotic-Induced Hyperprolactinemia:
- Reduce medication dosage.
- Switch to another antipsychotic agent.
- Administer low doses of dopamine agonists:
  √ Cabergoline (0.5 mg IM weekly).
  √ Quinagolide (0.025–0.075 mg/day).
  √ Bromocriptine (2.5–7.5 mg bid).
    □ Side effects (nausea, dizziness, headache) make this medication difficult to tolerate.

- Begin an oral contraceptive.
  √ Restores estrogen and thereby offers protection against the long-term adverse effects of a hypoestrogenic state.
  √ Hyperprolactinemic patients receiving estrogen should be monitored for signs/symptoms of an expanding prolactinoma.
    □ Headache.
    □ Visual loss.
    □ Cranial neuropathies.
    □ Further elevation in prolactin.
  √ If an undiagnosed prolactinoma is present, estrogen supplementation may increase its size.

Extrapyramidal Symptoms (EPS)

- Relatively common side effect of conventional antipsychotics.
- Akinesia (stiffness) seen in up to 50% of treated patients.
  √ May resemble negative symptoms.
  √ May be associated with higher rates of depression, anhedonia.
  √ Treated effectively with anticholinergic agents.
- Akathisia (motor restlessness) seen in up to 25% of treated patients.
  √ Twice as common in women.
  √ May resemble agitation/anxiety.
  √ Treated by lowering dose or by adding beta-blockers, anticholinergic agents, or benzodiazepines.
- Dystonia (sudden muscle contraction), typically of jaw.
  √ Treated quickly and effectively by parenteral anticholinergic medication (e.g., benztropine) or diphenhydramine.
- Oculogyric crisis (involuntary upward gaze)
- Tremor:
  √ Treated by lowering dose or by adding beta-blockers, anticholinergic agents, or benzodiazepines.

Tardive Dyskinesia (TD)

- Movement disorder associated with prolonged exposure to dopamine blockers, such as antipsychotics.
- Some but not all studies of TD in men and women have found greater prevalence in women, particularly women over age 50.
- Some studies have found that TD decreases with estrogen administration.
- Concern about tardive dyskinesia reflects its potential irreversibility.

- Characterized by hyperkinetic movements, worsening with stress, and disappearing during sleep.
- Most common forms:
  - √ Oral—chewing or tongue movements.
  - √ Extremities—choreoathetoid movements of fingers or, less commonly, toes.
- Less common forms:
  - √ Blepharospasm (involuntary closing of eyelids).
  - √ Truncal—with pelvic thrusting.
  - √ Respiratory.
- Must be distinguished (with great difficulty) from the spontaneous dyskinesias seen with schizophrenic patients not exposed to antipsychotics.
- Course is variable.
  - √ Does not universally progress, even with continued antipsychotic exposure.

Prevalence
- With conventional antipsychotics:
  - √ Patients < age 45 years: Risk is 4%/year for first five years (20% after 5 years).
    - □ Risk subsequently diminishes.
  - √ Patients > age 45 years: Risk is 29% after 1 year and 63% after 3 years.
- With risperidone and olanzapine:
  - √ Rate estimated to be one-quarter to one-tenth of that seen with conventional agents.
- Rate likely to be very low with quetiapine.
- Rate lowest with clozapine.

Major Risk Factors for Tardive Dyskinesia
- Duration of antipsychotic exposure.
- Type of antipsychotic (conventional antipsychotics confer higher risk).
- Female gender.
- Age: Marked increase for patients over age 45 years.
- Presence of EPS.
- Diabetes mellitus.
- Dose (higher dose confers higher risk).
- Intermittent dosing.
- Diagnosis (patients with mood disorders at higher risk).

Treatment of Tardive Dyskinesia
- No well-validated treatments.
- Switch to atypical antipsychotic if patient is on a conventional agent.
- If tardive dyskinesia is severe and socially impairing, consider switching to clozapine.
- Add vitamin E up to 1600 mg/day.
  - √ Data on efficacy are inconsistent.
- Add low-dose benzodiazepines.
  - √ May suppress dyskinesias somewhat.

PHASES OF TREATMENT

Acute

- Approximately first 8–12 weeks of treatment.
- Response rates may be higher with atypical agents.
- Response to antipsychotics is frequently partial rather than complete.
  - √ Residual psychotic symptoms remain in 40–50% of patients, even after 8–12 weeks of treatment.
- Rate of nonresponders in acute treatment ranges from 8 to 30%.

Continuation

- No clear guidelines exist for length of antipsychotic treatment (or dosage) after psychotic episode.
- After a single episode of schizophrenia, 12–18 months of antipsychotic treatment is generally recommended (based on clinical experience, not research data).

Maintenance

- Antipsychotics are more effective than placebo in reducing psychotic relapse.
- Rate of relapse with conventional antipsychotics: 53% for placebo vs. 16% for antipsychotic over 10 months.
- Long-term relapse rates are substantial even for closely-monitored patients.
- Atypical antipsychotics are associated with slightly lower relapse rates than conventional agents.

- All atypical agents appear comparable in preventive efficacy (with the possible exception of clozapine).
- Chronic schizophrenic patients (i.e., those with multiple relapses) should be recommended for maintenance treatment.
- Maintenance treatment is recommended after a single episode, but some single-episode patients may be slowly withdrawn from antipsychotics after 1 year if they are subsequently followed carefully.

TREATMENT CONSIDERATIONS FOR WOMEN OF REPRODUCTIVE AGE

- Obtain initial menstrual history.
  - √ Typical cycle length.
  - √ Typical duration of menses.
- Instruct patient to chart menstrual cycles after initiating treatment (e.g., with chart such as Figure 7.1), especially after initiating prolactin-elevating antipsychotic medications.
- Monitor patient's symptoms in relation to menstrual cycle.
  - √ If patient experiences recurrent premenstrual relapse or exacerbation of schizophrenia, consider increasing medication dose by 50% at midcycle.
- For heterosexual women who take antipsychotic medications and are sexually active:
  - √ If recent unprotected sex, obtain immediate pregnancy test.
  - √ OTC pregnancy tests are 99% accurate at 12–14 days postconception.
  - √ Educate about risks to fetus of medication exposure if patient becomes pregnant.
  - √ Encourage patient to use contraception regularly if she does not wish to conceive.
- Consider obtaining assessments of weight in medication management visits.
  - √ Medication-induced weight gain may lead to noncompliance with treatment.
  - √ Weight gain is associated with adverse health consequences, including hypertension, hyperlipidemia, and diabetes.
  - √ In women who conceive, obesity is linked with an increased risk of neural tube defects.

√ BMI (body mass index): weight in kg divided by height in meters, squared):
  □ BMI of 25–29.9: overweight.
  □ BMI of 30 or more: obese.

TREATMENT OF SCHIZOPHRENIA DURING PREGNANCY

* No antipsychotic agent currently has FDA approval for use during pregnancy.
* FDA use-in-pregnancy categories for medications are listed in Table 1.4.
* FDA use-in-pregnancy ratings for antipsychotic agents are listed in Table 6.7. Use in pregnancy ratings for additional medications are listed in Table 1.5.
* The decision to use an antipsychotic during pregnancy ultimately depends on:
  √ The risks of continued schizophrenic condition on the mother and fetus.
  √ Research findings on the safety/risks of medication use in pregnancy.
* Perform and record a careful risk–benefit discussion (see Table 1.3).

Table 6.7. Food and Drug Administration Use-in-Pregnancy Ratings for Certain Antipsychotic and Anticholinergic Medications

Medication	FDA Rating
Antipsychotics	
aripiprazole (Abilify)	C
chlorpromazine (Thorazine)	C
clozapine (Clozaril)	B
fluphenazine (Prolixin)	C
haloperidol (Haldol)	C
olanzapine (Zyprexa)	C
risperidone (Risperdal)	C
quetiapine (Seroquel)	C
trifluoperazine (Stelazine)	C
ziprasidone (Geodon)	C
Anticholinergic Agents	
benztropine (Cogentin)	C
diphenhydramine (Benadryl)	B
hydroxyzine (Atarax)	C
trihexyphenidyl (Artane)	C

SCHIZOPHRENIA

Use of Antipsychotic Agents in Pregnancy

- No adequate, well-controlled studies have examined the safety of antipsychotic agents during pregnancy.
- A significant limitation of many reports on the use of antipsychotic medications in pregnancy is that they involve small doses of medication used to treat nausea or insomnia, rather than the doses typically used for schizophrenia.

Phenothiazines

(For example, chlorpromazine [Thorazine], fluphenazine [Prolixin] trifluoperazine [Stelazine])

- Neonatal jaundice may occur following prenatal exposure to phenothiazines.
- First-trimester exposure to low-potency phenothiazines (in particular, those containing a 3-carbon aliphatic side chain; e.g., chlorpromazine) linked with a slight increase in the risk of nonspecific congenital malformations.
- When used near term, chlorpromazine has been linked with:
  - √ Neonatal respiratory distress.
  - √ Cyanosis.
  - √ Transient syndrome of tremor, hypotonia, and hyperreflexia.
- Exposure to prochlorperazine (a rarely-used phenothiazine) has been linked with increased height in children in one study.
  - √ Possibly a result of the medication's effect on growth hormone levels.
- Trifluoperazine and fluphenazine have been studied the most in pregnancy and do not appear to increase the risk for congenital malformations.
  - √ Most studies have been small, retrospective, and uncontrolled.

Haloperidol (Haldol)

- Two case reports described limb defects when haloperidol was used in the first trimester.
- One study of birth outcomes among 199 children of schizophrenic mothers reported a slightly elevated risk of nonspecific malformations among 29 children exposed to haloperidol in first trimester.
  - √ 10.3% vs. 2.5% among sample as a whole.
- Other reports, including a study of 100 exposures, did not identify a greater risk of congenital malformations in exposed infants.

Olanzapine (Zyprexa)

- Approximately 30 published exposures.
- Rates of spontaneous abortion, stillbirth, malformation, and prematurity have been within normal range.
- Because olanzapine use is associated with new-onset diabetes mellitus (see p. 137), its use during pregnancy theoretically may increase the risk for gestational diabetes.
  √ No reports have described this association to date.

Clozapine (Clozaril)

- Five published reports of prenatal exposures.
- No reports of congenital malformations.
- One case reported a seizure in an 8-day old baby who was exposed to clozapine in utero.

Risperidone (Risperdal)

- Two case reports showed no adverse outcomes in newborns.

Quetiapine (Seroquel)

- Two case reports showed no adverse outcomes in newborns.

Ziprasidone (Geodon), Aripiprazole (Abilify)

- No human studies are currently available on the use of these medications during pregnancy.

Agents to Treat Antipsychotic-Induced Extrapyramidal Side Effects

Trihexyphenidyl (Artane), Benztropine (Cogentin)

- Linked to miscellaneous minor congenital malformations and anticholinergic side effects in newborns, including:
  √ Bowel obstruction.
  √ Urinary retention.

Diphenhydramine (Benadryl)

- Linked with cleft lip in one case report, but generally appears safe to use in pregnancy.
- Linked with sedation and anticholinergic side effects in newborns.

S
C
H
I
Z
O
P
H
R
E
N
I
A

Propanolol (Inderal)

- No evidence of congenital malformations.
- Linked with neonatal bradycardia in one report.

Amantadine (Symmetrel)

- Linked with neonatal cardiovascular malformations in one case report.

Treatment Recommendations

- For women requiring an antipsychotic medication during pregnancy, reasonable choices are:
  √ Olanzapine.
  √ Trifluoperazine.
  √ Haloperidol.
- Use the minimum dose necessary.
- Minimize the use of agents to treat extrapyramidal side effects.

Antipsychotic Considerations Prior to Conception

If patient is likely to remain well off antipsychotics for at least a few weeks—e.g., if the antipsychotic medication is used for an episodic rather than chronic condition, such as bipolar disorder—and she is likely to conceive quickly (i.e., she is healthy, < age 35 years, with no history of infertility in herself or her partner):

- Try to taper and discontinue the antipsychotic medication before the patient attempts to conceive.
- Educate the patient about ways to maximize chances of conception by using methods to detect ovulation (e.g., by monitoring basal body temperature or using an OTC ovulation detection kit).

If the patient is likely to remain well off the antipsychotic for at least a few weeks, and she is NOT likely to conceive quickly:

- Continue the antipsychotic medication until patient has a positive pregnancy test (typically 14 days postconception, if patient performs a pregnancy test on the first day of her missed menstrual period).
- Once the patient is pregnant—and if she remains psychiatrically stable—taper and discontinue the medication.

√ The uteroplacental circulation begins forming at approximately 2 weeks postconception.
√ Therefore, the embryo generally receives minimal exposure.
√ OTC pregnancy tests turn positive at 12–14 days postconception.

If the risk of inadequately treated illness outweighs the potential risks associated with prenatal use of an antipsychotic medication— e.g., the patient has a history of severe relapses of schizophrenia following previous attempts at medication discontinuation:

- Continue the antipsychotic during pregnancy.
- Olanzapine, trifluoperazine, or haloperidol are reasonable choices.

TREATMENT OF SCHIZOPHRENIA DURING BREAST-FEEDING

- Little is known about the safety of antipsychotic medications during breast-feeding.
- Case reports of olanzapine and risperidone have noted no adverse effects in nursing infants.
- The median nursing infant's medication dose has been reported at approximately 1.6% of the weight-adjusted maternal dose for olanzapine; 4% for risperidone.
- A small study of haloperidol and chlorpromazine use during breast-feeding reported developmental delay in children exposed to high maternal doses of haloperidol (20–40 mg/day) in association with chlorpromazine.
  √ Study did not control for potentially confounding variables.
- Because data on the use of antipsychotics during breast-feeding are extremely limited, women should be advised not to breast-feed while on these medications.

Treatment Considerations for Breast-Feeding Patients Who Initiate Antipsychotic Medications

- Choose medications for which safety data exist on their use during breast-feeding.
- Prescribe the minimum dosage of medication that produces remission of symptoms.

SCHIZOPHRENIA

- Consider supplementation with bottle-feeding to reduce infant's medication exposure.
- Monitor the infant following the mother's initiation of the medication.
- Attempt to establish the infant's behavior, sleep and feeding patterns before beginning the medication.
  - √ Provides a baseline by which to determine whether the infant experiences adverse effects (e.g., decreased appetite, increased sleepiness) from medication exposure.
- Serum concentrations of medication do not need to be obtained routinely in infants, but the data may provide reassurance for some mothers.
- To obtain an infant serum concentration of medication:
  - √ Wait until medication serum levels are likely to be at steady state (i.e., at least five half-lives).
  - √ Ask the laboratory to use a high-sensitivity assay (i.e., with limit of detection < 2 ng/ml).
  - √ Measure concentrations of both the parent drug and its metabolites in infant serum.
  - √ At present, no cutoff point has been established for concern over serum concentrations of antidepressant medications in infant serum.
- Infants who are premature (< 36 weeks gestation) or have hepatic dysfunction should generally not be exposed to antipsychotic medications through breast milk.

TREATMENT CONSIDERATIONS FOR PERI- AND POSTMENOPAUSAL WOMEN

- Estrogen supplementation has been reported in some studies to:
  - √ Reduce negative symptoms.
  - √ Reduce the dosage of antipsychotic medication required for treatment.
  - √ Improve tardive dyskinesia.
- Additionally, some studies have reported:
  - √ Need for higher antipsychotic doses in postmenopausal women than in younger women.
  - √ Greater prevalence of tardive dyskinesia in women over age 50
  - √ Worse treatment response among postmenopausal women than premenopausal women, regardless of chronicity.

TREATMENT CONSIDERATIONS FOR ELDERLY WOMEN

- See Chapter 1, pages 18–19.
- The likelihood that women will develop tardive dyskinesia from antipsychotic agents rises with age.
- The likelihood of clozapine-associated agranulocytosis rises with age.

STRATEGIES FOR TREATMENT RESISTANCE

- No well-validated approaches available.
- For positive symptoms:
  - √ Switch to clozapine: Consider clozapine after two (or three) unsuccessful antipsychotic trials at adequate dose.
  - √ Combine two or more antipsychotics (a commonly used strategy but not well-studied).
  - √ Use two atypical agents, a conventional agent plus atypical, or clozapine plus atypical agent.
  - √ Add lithium—but results are generally poor.
  - √ Add valproate—one recent study showed positive results.
- For negative symptoms:
  - √ Begin an anticholinergic agent.
  - √ Negative symptoms may simply represent unrecognized drug-induced akinesia.
  - √ Begin an antidepressant (e.g., SSRI, mirtazapine).
    - □ Negative symptoms may simply represent unrecognized depression.
  - √ Add a dopamine agonist
    - □ d-amphetamine or modafanil: Use with caution because they may exacerbate psychosis.
    - □ Selegiline: Use low dose (5–10 mg/day); less likely to exacerbate psychosis.
    - □ Bupropion.
  - √ Switch to clozapine.

Neuroleptic Malignant Syndrome (NMS)

- Uncommon side effect, characterized by rigidity, hyperthermia, and autonomic instability, usually with high serum CPK (creatinine kinase) level.

S
C
H
I
Z
O
P
H
R
E
N
I
A

- May be seen in association with any antipsychotics.
- Prevalence rate < 1%.
- Risk factors include:
  √ Rapid dosing.
  √ High-potency conventional agents.
  √ Intramuscular administration.
  √ Dehydration.
  √ Preexisting neurological disorder.
- Women are at lower risk than men.
- May be fatal in up to 10% of cases.
- Treatment:
  √ Stop antipsychotic immediately.
  √ Hospitalize medically.
  √ Begin supportive measures.
  √ Consider dantrolene, bromocriptine (although neither has been well-studied for NMS).

7. Premenstrual Dysphoric Disorder

INTRODUCTION

Many women of reproductive age experience occasional physical and/or emotional symptoms in the days immediately preceding the onset of menses, colloquially referred to as "PMS." However, only a minority of women (approximately 5%) suffer from premenstrual dysphoric disorder (PMDD)—i.e., from symptoms that are severe enough to produce impairment in their daily functioning. PMDD refers to recurrent depression, anxiety, or irritability in the luteal phase of the menstrual cycle (i.e., following ovulation), with full remission after onset of menses. Women may also experience physical symptoms such as cramping, bloating, breast tenderness, and headaches.

Following the onset of menses, women often experience a dramatic improvement in their mood, sometimes to the point of elation. This mood shift can occur over the course of a single day or even over a few hours. This sharp switch in mood state can be mistaken for bipolar II disorder. Clinicians should be sure to screen for PMDD in women whom they believe to have bipolar II disorder, particularly if the patient experiences monthly depressions followed by apparent hypomanic episodes.

The biological etiology of PMDD has not yet been established. It is highly likely, however, that hormonal factors are implicated, given that the syndrome occurs only in menstruating women. Prepubertal girls and pregnant and menopausal women do not experience the syndrome. Research has evaluated the role of several hormones, including estrogen, progesterone, follicle-stimulating hormone (FSH), luteinizing hormone (LH), cortisol, dihydrotestosterone, and thyroid hormones, but none has been conclusively linked with the syndrome. A new and promising line of research is exploring the role of allo-pregnanolone, a metabolite of progesterone that has GABA-enhancing properties.

PMDD is not recognized as a discrete diagnostic category. In the *DSM-IV*, it is listed under "Mood Disorders Not Otherwise Specified." The criteria for PMDD are listed in Appendix A of the diagnostic manual under "Proposed Diagnostic Categories Needing Further Study." PMDD is the only disorder in the *DSM-IV* that requires prospective assessments before the diagnosis can be made. These assessments must be obtained over a minimum of two menstrual cycles. Given that these assessments entail postponing treatment for 2 months or longer, many clinicians initiate treatment on the basis of a patient's retrospective report of symptoms. After beginning treatment, patients should maintain a daily log of their emotional and physical symptoms to confirm that the symptoms are limited to the premenstrual phase of the cycle and to assess whether they are improving. Many patients find that the use of these daily logs gives them a reassuring sense of predictability regarding the onset of their symptoms.

EVALUATION OF WOMEN PRESENTING WITH PREMENSTRUAL DYSPHORIC DISORDER

- Screen for chronic psychiatric disorders.
  - √ Approximately two-thirds of women presenting for treatment of PMDD in fact suffer from premenstrual exacerbation of major depression, dysthymia, or an anxiety disorder.
  - √ If possible, women should be evaluated during the follicular phase of the menstrual cycle—i.e., the first 2 weeks after onset of menses. If a woman has PMDD, she should be symptom-free during this phase.
- Ask about a premenstrual increase in the use of alcohol or other substances (as potential attempts to self-medicate premenstrual symptoms).
- Ask about usual timing of symptoms.
  - √ Symptoms can last anywhere from the day prior to onset of menses to the entire 2-week duration of the luteal phase (beginning at midcycle, immediately after ovulation).

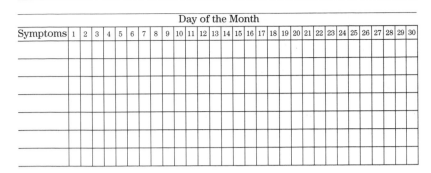

1. Circle days of period.
2. Rate symptom level of discomfort each day: 0 = Not at all;
   1 = Mild; 2 = Moderate; 3 = Severe.
3. Chart severity of symptoms.

Figure 7.1. Chart for Daily Symptom Ratings.

- Ideally, obtain daily symptom ratings (using chart such as shown in Figure 7.1) to confirm the diagnosis.
- Obtain a medical history and consider referring patient for a full physical and pelvic examination to screen for conditions that may worsen premenstrually and that present with symptoms that overlap with those of PMDD, including migraine headaches, endometriosis, chronic fatigue syndrome, fibromyalgia, fibrocystic breast disease, and irritable bowel syndrome.
- Consider obtaining laboratory measures to exclude other disorders. Specifically:
  √ If patient reports irregular menstrual cycles, obtain prolactin and thyroid function tests.
    □ Hyperprolactinemia and hypothyroidism can produce irregular menstrual cycles as well as changes in mood.
  √ If patient reports premenstrual fatigue, obtain thyroid function tests and a complete blood count to rule out hypothyroidism and anemia.
  √ If patient is over age 40 and reports irregular menstrual bleeding and/or hot flashes, obtain FSH and estradiol levels (see Chapter 1).
- Ask about the patient's dietary habits.
  √ Caffeine can exacerbate premenstrual headaches.
  √ Alcohol can exacerbate premenstrual fatigue.
  √ Salt can exacerbate premenstrual bloating.
  √ Inadequate consumption of certain vitamins and minerals

(vitamin B, vitamin E, calcium, magnesium) may exacerbate premenstrual symptoms.
- Ask about use of hormonal contraception.
  √ Certain forms of hormonal contraception may produce negative mood changes prior to the onset of menses.
  √ These premenstrual mood symptoms do not represent PMDD, because they are induced by exogenous hormones.
  √ Triphasic oral contraceptive preparations (in which hormone concentrations vary each week) are associated with greater variability in mood across the menstrual cycle, compared with monophasic preparations (in which hormones are maintained at steady concentrations) (see Table 9.4).
  √ Certain variables increase the likelihood that a woman will experience negative mood changes from hormonal contraception:
    □ History of PMDD.
    □ History of major depression.
    □ Family history of hormonal contraceptive-related depressive symptoms.
    □ A high level of emotional distress prior to initiating the hormonal contraceptive.
- If patient reports several premenstrual symptoms, ask her to identify which is most distressing. This information helps guide treatment.

TREATMENTS FOR PREMENSTRUAL DYSPHORIC DISORDER

Medication doses and timing of administration are listed in Table 7.1.

Antidepressants

- Antidepressants are highly effective for PMDD, regardless of whether the predominant symptom is depression, anxiety, or irritability.
- Best studied treatments: SSRIs.
- Venlafaxine, nefazodone, and tricyclic antidepressants also appear effective.
- Bupropion does not appear to be effective.
- Dosages are similar to those used for treatment of major depression (although some patients may respond to low doses).

Table 7.1. Pharmacological Treatments of Premenstrual Dysphoric Disorder

Medication	Dosage	When Administered
Antidepressants		
citalopram	20–40 mg/day	Throughout cycle, or midcycle to onset of menses
fluoxetine	10–20 mg/day	Throughout cycle, or midcycle to onset of menses
sertraline	50–100 mg/day	Throughout cycle, or midcycle to onset of menses
paroxetine	10–30 mg/day	Throughout cycle, or midcycle to onset of menses
clomipramine	25–75 mg/day	Throughout cycle
nortriptyline	50–100 mg/day	Throughout cycle
venlafaxine	75–375 mg/day	Throughout cycle
nefazodone	100–600 mg/day	Throughout cycle
Stimulants		
dextroamphetamine	10–20 mg/day	Symptomatic days
Anxiolytics		
alprazolam	0.25–5 mg/day	Symptomatic days
buspirone	15–60 mg/day	Throughout cycle or symptomatic days
Hormones		
estradiol implants	50–100 mg	Every 4–7 months subcutaneously
estradiol patches	2 patches @ 100 mcg	Every 3 days
oral micronized progesterone	200–1200 mg/day	Luteal phase
vaginal progesterone	200 mg suppositories bid	Luteal phase
leuprolide	3.75 mg	Every 4 weeks intramuscularly
danazol	200–400 mg	Midcycle to onset of menses
Oral Contraceptives		
yasmin	n/a	Daily
Diuretics		
spironolactone	25 mg qid	Symptomatic days
hydrochlorothiazide	25–50 mg/day	Symptomatic days
dyazide	1 capsule	Symptomatic days
Prostaglandin Inhibitors		
ibuprofen	600 mg bid–tid	Symptomatic days
mefenamic acid	250–500 mg tid	Symptomatic days
naproxen sodium	500 mg bid	Symptomatic days
Vitamins/Minerals		
vitamin E	400 IU/day	Throughout cycle
pyridoxine	50–100 mg/day	Throughout cycle
calcium	500 mg bid	Throughout cycle
magnesium	360 mg tid	Midcycle to onset of menses

(cont.)

Table 7.1. *Continued*

Medication	Dosage	When Administered
	Antihypertensives	
clonidine	17 μg/kg/day	Throughout cycle
atenolol	50 mg/day	Throughout cycle
propanolol	10–20 mg tid	Symptomatic days
	Miscellaneous	
bromocriptine	2.5 mg bid–tid	Day 10 to onset of menses
evening primrose oil	1–4 g/day	Midcycle to onset of menses
naltrexone	25 mg bid	Days 9–18 of cycle
gingko biloba	40–80 mg tid	Throughout cycle

- For antidepressant side effects, see Chapter 3.
- SSRI antidepressants have been reported effective when taken either on a daily basis or during the luteal phase of the cycle (from midcycle to onset of menses).
  √ This approach should not be recommended to women with irregular menstrual cycles (they will not consistently know when their luteal phase begins).
- Premenstrual somatic complaints (e.g., cramping, breast tenderness) also may improve with antidepressants.
- Treatment response to antidepressants occurs quickly, often within a few days.

Anxiolytics

- For women with primarily premenstrual anxiety and irritability, alprazolam and buspirone can be used.
- For side effects, see Chapter 5.

Stimulants

- Dextroamphetamine is helpful for women whose primary complaint is premenstrual fatigue.
- For side effects, see pages 66–68.

Hormonal Strategies

- Synthetic progestins (e.g., medroxyprovera) do not appear to be effective.
- Natural progesterone:

√ Formulations include:
  □ Oral micronized progesterone, 200–1200 mg/day.
  □ Vaginal progesterone 200 mg suppositories twice daily.
√ Taken during the luteal phase of the menstrual cycle.
√ Generally does not appear to be effective for PMDD in most studies.
√ However, may help a subgroup of women whose symptoms consist predominantly of premenstrual anxiety, tension, or irritability.
  □ Researchers speculate that the metabolites of natural progesterone (pregnanolone and allopregnanolone), which enhance GABA, may produce these anxiolytic effects.
√ Side effects of progesterone include increased appetite, weight gain, fatigue, and decreased libido.

- Estrogen:
  √ Effectively treats premenstrual psychological and physical symptoms, probably as a result of suppression of the hypothalamic–pituitary–ovarian axis.
  √ Prolonged estrogen use (> 3 months) is not recommended.
    □ Associated with uterine hyperplasia and increased risk of breast cancer.
  √ Side effects of estrogen include nausea, breast tenderness, and weight gain.
- Gonadotropin-releasing hormone (GnRH) agonists:
  √ Include leuprolide (Lupron), nafarelin (Synarel), and goserelin (Zoladex).
  √ Suppress the hypothalamic–pituitary–ovarian axis and are effective for PMDD.
  √ However, they produce an anovulatory (and therefore hypoestrogenic) state, which may lead to hot flashes, vaginal dryness, and loss of bone mass.
  √ With long-term therapy (> 6 months), osteopenia and/or osteoporosis can occur.
  √ To minimize hypoestrogenic and osteopenic effects, hormonal add-back therapy should be implemented; however, premenstrual symptoms may recur.
  √ GnRH agonists not recommended for long-term use.
- Hormonal contraception:
  √ Oral contraceptives are generally of little benefit for premenstrual mood symptoms but can help reduce premenstrual physical symptoms.

√ Exception: Yasmin (drospirenone/ethinyl estradiol): new birth control pill that appears effective for premenstrual mood and physical symptoms. It contains a novel progestin (drospirenone) with antimineralocorticoid and antiandrogenic activity.

Vitamins and Minerals

- Well tolerated but inconsistently effective.
- Pyridoxine (vitamin B_6).
  √ Doses should not exceed 100 mg/day (higher doses can produce peripheral neuropathy).
- Calcium.
- Magnesium.
- Vitamin E.

Diuretics

- E.g., spironolactone, dyazide.
- Helpful for discomfort associated with premenstrual fluid retention.
- Helpful for mood symptoms in women with significant premenstrual fluid retention.
- Need to be taken only during symptomatic days.
- Hypokalemia, dizziness, and orthostasis are potential side effects.

Prostaglandin Inhibitors

- Prostaglandins are naturally occurring substances involved in inflammatory responses.
- Prostaglandin inhibitors can help reduce pain and swelling and include:
  √ Ibuprofen (e.g., Motrin).
  √ Mefenamic acid (e.g., Ponstel).
  √ Naproxen sodium (e.g., Anaprox, Naprosyn).
- Helpful for pain, headaches, and cramping.
- Not helpful for mood symptoms.
- Work most effectively if started before the onset of symptoms (e.g., 7–10 days prior to menses) and taken as needed thereafter.

Miscellaneous Agents

- Beta-blockers (e.g., atenolol, propanolol) and clonidine are helpful for premenstrual irritability and anxiety.
- The opiate antagonist naltrexone has been reported to reduce miscellaneous premenstrual physical and psychological symptoms.
- Gingko biloba has been reported to help breast tenderness and bloating.
- Evening primrose oil may help, but evidence for its efficacy is inconsistent.
- Danazol, a synthetic androgen, suppresses the hypothalamic–pituitary–ovarian axis and therefore effectively treats PMDD.
  √ Produces significant side effects, including acne, weight gain, and hirsutism.

Nonpharmacological Treatments

- Exercise.
- Stress reduction in the premenstrual phase of the menstrual cycle.
- Relaxation techniques.
- Education.
- Acupuncture.
- Dietary modification:
  √ Reduce caffeine, alcohol, nicotine.
  √ Consume foods rich in vitamin B, vitamin E, calcium, and magnesium.

Treatment Considerations

- For mild premenstrual depression or anxiety (PMS or mild PMDD), consider vitamins, minerals, and beta-blockers.
- Treat physical symptoms (e.g., cramping, bloating), if any, and mood is likely to improve (at least somewhat).
- For all patients, encourage nonpharmacological interventions, including exercise and stress reduction, in the premenstrual phase of the menstrual cycle.
- During treatment, patients should keep a daily log of their mood so that treatment efficacy can be adequately assessed.
- Continue a treatment trial for at least two menstrual cycles to assess its efficacy.

PREMENSTRUAL DYSPHORIC DISORDER

- For moderate or severe symptoms, antidepressant medications are reasonable first-line treatments.
- In choosing an antidepressant medication, consider:
  - √ Patient's preferred treatment schedule (continuous vs. luteal phase only).
    - □ SSRIs (but, to date, no other antidepressants) can be prescribed either in luteal phase or daily.
  - √ Plans regarding pregnancy.
    - □ If patient plans to conceive in near future, try to use medications with safety data in pregnancy.
  - √ Additional factors to consider are listed in Chapter 3 (pp. 35–36).
- If patient fails the first antidepressant trial, switch to a second antidepressant.
- If two or three antidepressants are tried without success, review the diagnosis and consider an alternative treatment approach (e.g., hormonal strategy, stimulant, anxiolytic).
- The length of pharmacological treatment for PMDD has not been well-established; most likely, treatment should continue as long as patient continues to ovulate.
  - √ Some women may be able to discontinue treatment after long periods of stability.

8. Eating Disorders

Over 90% of cases of anorexia nervosa and bulimia nervosa occur in women. These illnesses typically develop during adolescence or early adulthood and affect approximately 1–3% of women. With treatment, 45–70% of patients eventually overcome these disorders, but a substantial proportion remain chronically ill. Anorexia nervosa tends to be more treatment-refractory than bulimia nervosa and is associated with a mortality rate of 5%. Fatalities result primarily from the medical sequelae of anorexia nervosa. In patients with comorbid major depression, suicide also contributes to the fatality rate.

Anorexia nervosa is categorized into two types: restricting type and binge-eating/purging type. Approximately 50% of cases of anorexia fall into each category. Bulimia nervosa is also categorized in two types: purging type (i.e., involving the use of self-induced vomiting, laxatives, diuretics, or enemas) and the more rarely seen nonpurging type (involving other forms of compensatory behaviors, e.g., excessive exercise or fasting).

Some studies have reported that risk factors for anorexia nervosa include perfectionism, a negative self-image, and participation in certain professions (e.g., professional dancing, modeling, and athletics). Risk factors for bulimia nervosa include depression, substance abuse, history of sexual and physical abuse, early menarche, obesity, low self-esteem, family conflict, parental obesity, and parental weight concern. Favorable prognostic factors for both anorexia nervosa and bulimia nervosa include young age of onset, short time between the onset of symptoms and treatment, less familial psychopathology, and absence of comorbid personality disorder. Cluster C (anxious/avoidant) personality traits are common in patients with anorexia nervosa, whereas Cluster B (dramatic/erratic, emotionally dysregulated) personality disorders (e.g., borderline personality disorder) are seen in a substantial minority (approximately 30%) of patients with bulimia nervosa.

Patients with bulimia nervosa are usually of normal weight and therefore the diagnosis can be easily missed. Women with eating disorders often feel ashamed of their eating behaviors and may be reluctant to disclose them, adding to the possibility of overlooked diagnoses. Clinicians working with female patients, particularly young women, should routinely inquire about eating habits, body image, actual and desired weight, menstrual patterns, exercise, self-induced vomiting, and use of laxatives, diuretics, enemas, emetics, diet pills, and stimulants. Women experiencing unexplained infertility also should be screened for eating disorders, in particular, anorexia nervosa.

Comorbid psychiatric disorders occur in up to 80% of patients with bulimia or anorexia nervosa. The most common comorbid disorders are depression, anxiety disorders, and substance and alcohol abuse.

Patients with eating disorders ideally should receive multidisciplinary care from a treatment team that includes mental health professionals, primary care physicians, and nutritionists. Clinicians can help build a therapeutic alliance if they acknowledge that treatment commonly produces great anxiety in patients—e.g., from fear of gaining weight or giving up their familiar eating patterns. Patients may try to "split" the team by misrepresenting what others have said or disparaging certain members of the team. Ongoing communication among the team members and agreement on key issues (e.g., the rate of weight gain expected of the patient) will help reduce this splitting and ultimately benefit the patient's progress.

Pharmacological treatments are somewhat helpful in treating the symptoms of bulimia nervosa, (e.g., binge-eating and self-induced purging) but are significantly less effective for the restrictive eating of anorexia nervosa. Therefore, nonpharmacological approaches are essential for the treatment of anorexia nervosa, including individual therapy, family therapy, and group support. Patients with bulimia nervosa also should be offered these approaches. Cognitive–behavioral therapy is a particularly well-researched and effective treatment for bulimia nervosa. Dialectical behavior therapy and interpersonal therapy also have been reported to help.

Binge-eating disorder (BED) is a newly-proposed diagnosis listed in the appendix of the *DSM-IV* as a condition requiring further study. Patients with this condition consume large amounts of food while feeling a loss of control over their eating. Unlike patients with bulimia nervosa, these patients do not engage in compensatory behaviors such as self-induced purging or excessive exercise. Many patients with BED are obese. The major complications of this disorder are the diseases that accompany obesity, including diabetes, high blood pressure, elevated cholesterol, and heart disease.

TREATMENT OF ANOREXIA AND BULIMIA NERVOSA

The priority in treatment is evaluation and stabilization of medical sequelae, if any, from the eating disorder (see Table 8.1).

* Persistently amenorrheic patients who are physically active (e.g., athletes) may additionally require a bone densitometry to screen for osteopenia and osteoporosis.
* Patients with eating disorders should be screened for mood, anxiety, and substance use disorders.
  √ These are common comorbidities.
  √ In many cases, mood and anxiety disorders remit following weight restoration.

Table 8.1. Potential Medical Complications of Anorexia and Bulimia Nervosa

Physiological System	Potential Complications
Cardiovascular	Electrocardiographic abnormalities (e.g., prolonged QT interval)
	Hypotension
	Sinus bradycardia
	Atrial and ventricular arrhythmias
Gastrointestinal	Esophageal perforation
	Gastric rupture
	Rectal prolapse
	Elevated serum amylase
Endocrine	Metabolic alkalosis
	Hypokalemia
	Amenorrhea
Bone	Osteoporosis
Orofacial	Erosion of dental enamel
	Parotid and submandibular gland hypertrophy
Hematologic	Anemia
	Thrombocytopenia
	Leukopenia

EATING DISORDERS

Table 8.2. Laboratory Evaluation of Patients with Anorexia and Bulimia Nervosa

Test	Purpose
Blood urea nitrogen Creatinine Electrolytes	To assess fluid and electrolyte abnormalities
Calcium Glucose Magnesium Phosphorus Liver function tests (including albumin and total protein)	To assess nutritional status
Complete blood count	To assess for anemia, leukopenia, thrombocytopenia
Reproductive hormones: luteinizing hormone (LH), follicle stimulating hormone (FSH), estradiol (E_2)	To evaluate for persistent (> 3 months) amenorrhea
Thyroid function tests	To assess thyroid status; may influence weight and appetite, menstrual cycling
Electrocardiogram	To assess for EKG abnormalities

PHARMACOLOGICAL TREATMENTS FOR BULIMIA NERVOSA AND BINGE-EATING DISORDER

- Patients with bulimia nervosa or binge-eating disorder can usually be managed in outpatient settings.
- Medications that affect fluid and electrolyte status, e.g., lithium, should be used very cautiously in patients with bulimia.

Antidepressant Medications

- Help reduce the frequency of binge-eating episodes, purging behavior, and depressive symptomatology in short-term treatment.
- May be effective even for patients without concomitant depression.
- The optimal duration of antidepressant treatment for bulimia nervosa has not been established.
- At present, long-term (indefinite) maintenance therapy is recommended, although the frequency of relapse appears high even among patients treated with maintenance antidepressants.

- Persistence is critical: Many patients fail the first trial but respond to subsequent antidepressant trials.
- The efficacy for bulimia nervosa appears similar across antidepressants (but data on this point are limited).
- A combination of antidepressants plus psychotherapy appears more effective at reducing binge frequency compared to antidepressants alone.
- Serotonin reuptake inhibitors:
  - √ Currently the most widely used agents for bulimia nervosa and binge-eating disorder.
  - √ Fluoxetine studied the most.
    - □ High doses (60–80 mg/day) appear more effective than lower doses (20 mg/day).
  - √ Other SSRIs are also likely to work.
  - √ For dosage and side effects, see Chapter 3.
- Tricyclic antidepressants:
  - √ Reported helpful for bulimia nervosa and binge-eating disorder.
  - √ Rarely used because of side effects and poor patient acceptability.
  - √ Desipramine and imipramine studied the most.
  - √ TCAs have the disadvantage of promoting weight gain.
  - √ Used at doses similar to those typically used to treat depression (see Chapter 3).
  - √ For side effects, see Chapter 3.
- Monoamine oxidase inhibitors:
  - √ Reported helpful for bulimia nervosa.
  - √ Phenelzine and isocarboxazid studied the most.
  - √ Hypertensive crisis can occur if patient ingests tyramine-containing foods (see Chapter 3).
  - √ These medications are generally problematic to use in a population of patients with little control over their eating.
- Bupropion:
  - √ Reported helpful for bulimia nervosa.
  - √ Not recommended for women at risk for electrolyte imbalance.
    - □ These women may be at increased risk for medication-induced seizures (black box warning about this risk).
  - √ Some clinicians use it for treatment-refractory cases but additionally use an antiepileptic drug (e.g., topiramate).

EATING DISORDERS

- Venlafaxine:
  √ Reported helpful for binge-eating disorder.
  √ For dosage and side effects, see Chapter 3.

Other Agents

- Topiramate:
  √ Reported helpful for bulimia nervosa and binge-eating disorder.
  √ Should be titrated up gradually to reduce dropout rate.
  √ For dosage and side effects, see Chapter 4.

PHARMACOLOGICAL TREATMENTS FOR ANOREXIA NERVOSA

- Following medical stabilization, treatment should focus on establishing regular and healthy eating.
- Most patients with anorexia nervosa require intensive treatment in an inpatient setting or day program, where they can be supported in eating and restoring their weight.
- Patients often try to circumvent treatment (e.g., by hiding and secretly throwing away food; holding food in their mouths until it can be disposed of), necessitating close monitoring.
- Consider hospitalizing patients if body weight is 25% below normal and patient experiences medical complications (see Table 8.1), refuses to eat, or fails to gain weight with outpatient treatment.
- Weight gain should proceed at 2–3 lbs./week for inpatients and ½–2 lbs/week for outpatients.
- Patients should be asked to remove jackets and empty pockets when being weighed.
  √ They may try to make their weight gain appear greater by carrying objects in their pockets or wearing heavy clothing.
- After symptoms improve, long-term maintenance therapy is recommended with either antidepressants or atypical antipsychotics.
- Use caution in prescribing medications that prolong QT interval or reduce blood pressure (e.g., antipsychotics, TCAs).
  √ QT interval is already prolonged in many patients with anorexia nervosa.

√ Patients with eating disorders often are hypotensive and may experience significant orthostasis.

Antidepressants

- Controlled trials have not found evidence that antidepressants help improve outcomes for anorexia nervosa.
- However, they may help maintain recovery after weight restoration.
- Antidepressants also may be helpful for comorbid mood and anxiety disorders, although their efficacy may be diminished in a low-weight state.

Atypical Antipsychotics

- Small studies have found olanzapine and risperidone to be helpful.
- For dosage and side effects, see Chapter 6.

TREATMENT OF EATING DISORDERS DURING PREGNANCY

- For many women with eating disorders, eating patterns become less disturbed during pregnancy.
- Women with eating disorders should be encouraged to put off pregnancy until they no longer have active symptoms.
- Eating disorders during pregnancy pose risks to the woman and fetus from:
  √ Electrolyte imbalance.
  √ Malnutrition.
  √ Inadequate weight gain.
  √ Preterm delivery.
- The treatment of eating disorders in pregnant women should include education about the importance of adequate nutrition and weight gain for the fetus.
- Warning signs suggestive of eating disorder in pregnancy:
  √ Inadequate weight gain.
  √ History of eating disorders.
  √ Hyperemesis gravidarum.
    □ Reported in approximately 10% of bulimic women, in contrast to the community prevalence of 1 in 1,000.

EATING DISORDERS

□ Bulimic patients may use the diagnosis to rationalize their self-induced vomiting.

□ It is probably wise for clinicians to consider an eating disorder whenever a pregnant patient reports recurrent hyperemesis gravidarum.

• Treatment with SSRIs or TCAs can be helpful for bulimia; choose agents with safety data in pregnancy (see Chapter 3).

• Consider increasing the frequency of nonpharmacological interventions (e.g., group support, individual psychotherapy) to minimize the need for medication during pregnancy.

• Women with eating disorders may feel more comfortable if their weight gain during pregnancy is not revealed to them at routine prenatal visits (unless the weight gain is inadequate).

TREATMENT OF EATING DISORDERS FOLLOWING DELIVERY

Postpartum Relapse of Eating Disorders

• Among patients with bulimia who become pregnant

√ Approximately 60% relapse following delivery, with bulimic behaviors often becoming worse than they were before conception.

√ Approximately 25–33% are no longer bulimic after the delivery.

√ Risk factors for relapse include

□ History of severe and persistent bulimia.

□ History of anorexia.

□ Unplanned pregnancy.

• Infant's weight gain should be monitored in the postpartum.

√ Some mothers with eating disorders become preoccupied with the infant's weight and make efforts to limit the infant's feeding.

• Compared to the general population of new mothers, women with eating disorders more commonly report difficulty with breast-feeding and premature termination of breast-feeding.

Postpartum Depression

• Women with bulimia nervosa face approximately a 30% risk of postpartum major depression.

- Women with anorexia nervosa face approximately a 60% risk of postpartum major depression.
- These risks are substantially higher than the 12–13% risk faced by new mothers in the general population.
- Factors that increase the risk for postpartum depression among women with eating disorders include active symptoms of the eating disorder during the pregnancy and high frequency of bingeing after delivery.
- Antidepressant medications can be prescribed to treat postpartum eating disorders as well as postpartum depression, even if the mother is breast-feeding. See Chapter 3 for details.

EATING DISORDERS

9. Female Reproductive Hormones and the Central Nervous System

REVIEW OF FEMALE ENDOCRINOLOGY

The female reproductive system is regulated by a complex ·interaction of hormones. In women of reproductive age, the menstrual cycle begins at the hypothalamus, where gonadotropin releasing hormone (GnRH) is released in a pulsatile fashion every 60–90 minutes. GnRH travels to the pituitary gland, where it stimulates the production of follicle-stimulating hormone (FSH) and luteinizing hormone (LH). These in turn stimulate the ovaries to produce ovarian follicles, which produce estradiol, the principal estrogen made by the ovaries. Approximately 3–30 follicles grow during this first half of the menstrual cycle, called the follicular phase (see Figure 9.1).

Over the course of 10–14 days, one ovarian follicle becomes dominant and the others degenerate. A midcycle surge in LH causes ovulation or release of the egg from the dominant ovarian follicle. Ovulation test kits measure this surge in LH. Ovulation occurs approximately 16–32 hours after the LH surge. An egg takes about 5 days to travel down the fallopian tube to the uterus.

Around the time of ovulation many women experience a dull pain in the lower abdomen, known as "*mittelschmerz*" (meaning, middle pain). The ruptured follicle becomes a corpus luteum ("yellow body") and produces progesterone, which prepares the uterine lining for implantation of a fertilized egg. This phase of the cycle is called the luteal

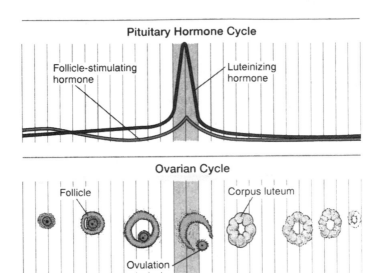

Pituitary Hormone Cycle

Follicle-stimulating hormone

Luteinizing hormone

Ovarian Cycle

Follicle

Corpus luteum

Ovulation

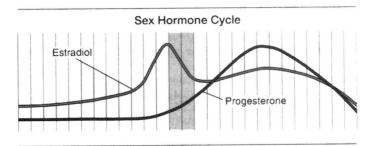

Sex Hormone Cycle

Estradiol

Progesterone

Endometrial Cycle

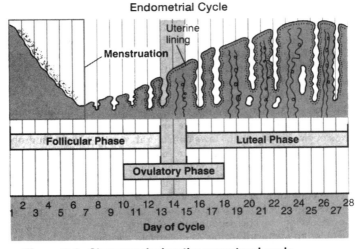

Uterine lining

Menstruation

Follicular Phase

Luteal Phase

Ovulatory Phase

1 2 3 4 5 6 7 8 9 10 11 12 13 14 15 16 17 18 19 20 21 22 23 24 25 26 27 28

Day of Cycle

Figure 9.1. Changes during the menstrual cycle.
(From *The Merck Manual of Medical Information—Home Edition,*
p. 1076, edited by Mark H. Beers and Robert Berkow. Copyright 1997
by Merck & Co., Inc., Whitehouse Station, NJ.)

phase. The rise in progesterone causes a woman's body temperature to increase. This rise in temperature can be used to monitor the timing of ovulation.

If a woman does not conceive, the corpus luteum degenerates after 14 days and progesterone production drops. The drop in progesterone leads to menstruation and the start of a new cycle. The length of the menstrual cycle ranges from 23 to 35 days. Only 10–15% of women have cycles that are exactly 28 days.

If the egg is fertilized, the corpus luteum produces human chorionic gonadotropin (HCG). This hormone maintains the corpus luteum and the production of progesterone, which are necessary for the pregnancy. Pregnancy tests are based on detecting increased levels of human chorionic gonadotropin. Once the placenta develops, it takes over the production of progesterone.

Menstrual cycles continue until women reach menopause. *Perimenopause* describes the transition between a woman's reproductive years and menopause. Perimenopause usually occurs between ages 40 to 55 (average age 47) and can last anywhere from a few months to several years. Perimenopausal women typically experience irregular menstrual cycles and symptoms of declining estrogen such as hot flashes and night sweats. These are sensations of intense heat typically lasting 2–3 minutes and varying widely in frequency from one woman to another. Some women experience these flashes several times a day whereas others rarely experience them. Declining estrogen also can produce vaginal dryness, loss of fullness in the breasts, and thinning hair.

To determine if a patient is perimenopausal, the FSH level should be obtained on day 2 or 3 after the onset of menstruation. FSH levels obtained at other times in the menstrual cycle can be inconclusive because they vary widely across the cycle. Once menstrual cycles have ceased for 12 months, a woman has reached menopause. Natural menopause occurs between ages 44 and 55 years (average age 51 years).

In addition to estrogen, the ovaries produce dehydroepiandrosterone (DHEA), dehydroepiandrosterone sulfate (DHEAS), and androstenedione, which are the predominant androgens in women. They are precursors in the synthesis of testosterone and estrone, the main estrogen found in postmenopausal women. DHEA and DHEAS are produced by the ovaries and adrenal glands and converted to testosterone and estrone in adipose tissue, muscle, and skin. At menopause, ovarian

Table 9.1. Average Serum Concentrations of Hormones in Adult Women

Estradiol, E2

Follicular	30–100 pg/ml
Ovulatory	100–400
Luteal	60–150
Pregnant	Up to 35,000
Postmenopausal	< 18

Progesterone

Follicular phase	0.2–1.4 ng/ml
Luteal phase	3.3–28
Postmenopausal	< 0.7
Pregnant	Up to 422

FSH

Follicular	2.5–10.2 mIU/ml
Ovulatory	3.4–33.4
Luteal	1.5–9.1
Perimenopausal	> 20–25
Postmenopausal	23–116.3
Pregnant	< 0.2

LH

Follicular	1.9–12.5 mIU/ml
Ovulatory	8.7–76.3
Luteal	0.5–16.9
Postmenopausal	5–52.3

Prolactin

Nonpregnant	2.8–29.2 ng/ml
Pregnant	9.7–208.5
Postmenopausal	1.8–20

Androgens*

Androstenedione	47–268 ng/ml
Dehydroepiandrosterone	60–995 ng/dL
Dehydroepiandrosterone sulfate	13–395 ng/dL
Testosterone	0.3–6.7 ng/dL

* Levels decline gradually with age.
(*Sources:* Yen SSC, Jaffe RB, Barbieri RL. *Reproductive Endocrinology: Physiology, Pathophysiology, and Clinical Management.* 4th edition. Philadelphia: WB Saunders; 1999. Laboratory Corporation of America, Burlington, North Carolina.)

production of androgens falls. Adrenal androgen production also falls with age, but this fall is age-related rather than menopause-related and therefore more gradual.

HORMONE SUPPLEMENTATION

Most women take exogenous hormones at some point in their lives. These are typically prescribed as hormonal contraceptives and as hormone replacement therapy. In the past two decades these hormonal supplements have become safer and better tolerated because of a

Table 9.2. Potential Estrogenic, Progestational, and Androgenic Side Effects

Hormone	Potential Side Effects
Estrogenic	Breast tenderness
	Nausea
	Weight gain
Progestational	Increased appetite
	Weight gain
	Fatigue
	Decreased libido
Androgenic	Hirsutism
	Acne
	Weight gain
	Lowering of voice
	Lowered HDL

reduction in the levels of hormones used. Nevertheless, certain risks and side effects continue to accompany their use. For oral contraceptives, side effects depend on their relative estrogenic, progestational, and androgenic effects (Table 9.2). Oral contraceptives slightly increase the risk of certain medical conditions, such as elevated blood pressure and blood clots. These risks are faced primarily by women who smoke, are over age 35, or who have hypertension or a history of blood clots. On the other hand, oral contraceptives are associated with certain health benefits, including a lower risk of ovarian cancer and iron-deficiency anemia. Also, they typically improve premenstrual physical symptoms, such as cramping and breast pain.

Approximately 50% of postmenopausal women use hormone replacement therapy (HRT; combination of estrogen plus progestin/progesterone) or estrogen replacement therapy (ERT) at some time. The prevalence of use is higher among younger postmenopausal women (< 49 years) than among older women (> 59 years). HRT, in particular the estrogen component, is highly effective at relieving vasomotor and urogenital symptoms. It also prevents bone loss and reduces the incidence of osteoporotic fractures. Additional benefits include lower risks of macular degeneration and colon cancer.

For many years, HRT was believed to protect against cardiovascular disease. However, the Women's Health Initiative, a large, federally funded study, recently reported a slight increase, rather than a decrease, in the incidence of heart attacks and strokes in the year after initiation of HRT. Postmenopausal women with established heart disease comprised the group at greatest risk for these cardiovascular events. Studies are currently in progress to determine the impact of HRT on the risk of cardiovascular events in women without preexisting heart disease. Also, the Women's Health Initiative is continuing with an estrogen-only arm to determine whether estrogen alone—without the progestin component—may produce more favorable cardiovascular outcomes.

An important consideration in the use of estrogen is the subsequent increased risk for endometrial hyperplasia and uterine cancer. Progestogens therefore are typically administered to counteract estrogen's effects on the uterine lining. "Progestogen" is an umbrella term for progesterone, which is natural, and progestins, which are synthetic. Progestogens are administered either continuously (every day of the month) or cyclically (at a higher dose, 10–14 days of each month). The cyclic regimen produces progestin-withdrawal bleeding, similar to a menstrual period. Women who have had a hysterectomy do not require a progestin in addition to estrogen.

A variety of formulations of HRT are available in the United States (Table 9.5). Of these, the most widely prescribed is conjugated equine estrogen (Premarin). The most widely prescribed progestin is medroxyprogesterone acetate (Provera). Many women prefer to use herbal remedies and/or phytoestrogens (estrogen-like chemicals in plants). Soy and soy products are high in phytoestrogens. However, their usefulness for menopausal symptoms is controversial. The efficacy of herbal remedies (e.g., black cohosh) for menopausal symptoms is also inconclusive.

Testosterone supplementation is sometimes used in combination with HRT. It is administered as methyltestosterone because testosterone is inactive if given orally. Testosterone's main advantage is an increase in libido. It also reduces vasomotor symptoms, thereby reducing the amount of estrogen necessary. However, its use is limited by its potential masculinizing effects (see Table 9.2).

HORMONES AND MOOD

Some researchers have proposed that estrogen and progesterone may influence mood through their effects in the central nervous system. Progesterone and estrogen receptors are present throughout the brain, including the hypothalamus and limbic system, two areas involved in regulating emotion and mood. Estrogen decreases monoamine oxidase (MAO) activity, thereby diminishing the degradation of

Table 9.3. Estrogens and Progestins Used in Oral Contraceptive Formulations

Estrogens
  Ethinyl estradiol
  Mestranol

Progestins
  Chlormadinone acetate
  Ethynodiol diacetate
  Desogestrel
  Drospirenone
  Gestodene
  Norethindrone
  Levonorgestrel
  Medroxyprogesterone acetate
  Megestrol acetate
  Norethynodrel
  Norgestimate
  Norgestrel

norepinephrine and serotonin and thus increasing their activity. Progesterone has the reverse impact on MAO. Allopregnanolone, a metabolite of progesterone, is a potent neuroactive steroid that modulates GABA receptors and may influence vulnerability to premenstrual tension.

The impact of hormonal supplementation on mood remains controversial. Several studies have examined the impact of oral contraceptives (OC) on mood, and have generally found no difference in mood among OC users versus nonusers, with some exceptions. Specifically, certain variables increase the likelihood that a woman will experience negative mood changes from OC:

• History of PMS.
• History of major depression.
• Family history of OC-related depressive symptoms.
• High level of emotional distress prior to initiating OC.

Triphasic preparations (in which hormone concentrations vary each week) are associated with greater variability in mood across the menstrual cycle, compared with monophasic preparations (in which hormones are maintained at steady concentrations; see Table 9.4).

A smaller but rapidly growing literature has examined the impact of hormone replacement therapy on mood. The research has primarily focused on the use of estrogen for the treatment of depression in perimenopausal women. Most of the clinical trials, however, have been

Table 9.4. Relative Estrogenic, Progestational, and Androgenic Activity of Certain Oral Contraceptives

Contraceptive Formulation	Estrogenic Activity	Progestational Activity	Androgenic Activity	Monophasic, Biphasic, or Triphasic
Alesse	+	+	+	Mono
Brevicon	++	+	+	Mono
Cyclessa	+	++	+	Tri
Demulen	+	+	+	Mono
Desogen	+	+	+/−	Mono
Estrostep	+	+	+	Tri
Genora	++	++	++	Mono
Jenest	++	++	++	Bi
Levlen	+	++	++	Mono
Levlite	+	+	+	Mono
Loestrin 1.5/30	+	+++	+++	Mono
Loestrin 1/20	+	++	++	Mono
Lo-Ovral	+	+	++	Mono
Mircette	+	+	+/−	Bi
Modicon	++	+	+	Mono
Nordette	+	+	+	Mono
Ovcon 1/50	++	+	+	Mono
Ovral	+++	+++	+++	Mono
Orthocept	+	+	+/−	Mono
Ortho-Novum 1/35	++	++	+	Mono
Ortho-Novum 7/7/7	++	+	+/−	Tri
Ortho-Tricyclen	++	++	+	Tri
Tri-Levlen	++	+	+/−	Tri
Triphasil	++	+	+/−	Tri
Yasmin	+	+	−	Mono

+/− None to minimal; + mild; ++ moderate; +++ significant.

uncontrolled or retrospective. Generally, the studies show that physiological doses of estrogen produce modest mood-elevating effects and may be helpful for mild depression. This effect is independent of estrogen's relief of vasomotor symptoms. Estrogen's efficacy for major depression, either as monotherapy or as an augmentation to antidepressants, is less compelling, although recent studies of estradiol for major depression (particularly mild cases) have shown promising results.

The psychiatric side effects associated with the use of medications to treat infertility (e.g., ovulation-inducing agents such as clomiphene) have received very little attention. Case reports have described mood swings, but systematic studies are lacking. Another question that remains to be further researched involves the impact of testosterone on mood in women. Preliminary data, which have documented a positive effect of testosterone on mood and well-being in postmenopausal women, appear to be promising.

Table 9.5. HRT Formulations and Dosages

Brand Name	Type of Hormone	Dose (mg)
	Oral Estrogen Preparations	
Premarin	Conjugated equine estrogen	0.3, 0.625, 0.9, 1.25, 2.5
Estrace	Micronized estradiol	0.5, 1, 2
Estratab	Esterified estrogen	0.3, 0.625, 2.5
Menest	Esterified estrogen	0.3, 0.625, 1.25, 2.5
Cenestin	Conjugated estrogen	0.625, 0.9, 1.25
Ortho-est	Estropipate	0.625, 1.25
Ogen	Estropipate	0.625, 1.25, 2.5
	Transdermal Estrogen Preparations	
Alora	Transdermal estrogen	1.5, 2.5, 3
Climara	Transdermal estrogen	0.05, 0.1
Estraderm	Transdermal estrogen	0.05, 0.1
Vivelle	Transdermal estrogen	0.0375, 0.05, 0.075, 0.1
	Vaginal Estrogens	
Estrace	Micronized estradiol	1.0
Ogen vaginal cream	Estropipate	1.5
Estring	Estradiol	2-mg reservoir
Vagifem	Estradiol	25 mcg
Ortho Dienestrol	Dienestrol	0.1%
Premarin vaginal cream	Conjugated equine estrogen	0.625
	Progestogen Preparations	
Amen	Medroxyprogesterone acetate	10
Cycrin	Medrogxyprogesterone acetate	2.5, 5, 10
Megace	Megestrol acetate	20, 40, 160
Micronor	Norethindrone	0.35
Nor-QD	Norethindrone	0.35
Aygestin	Norethindrone acetate	5
Ovrette	Norgestrel	0.075
	Progesterone	
Prometrium	Micronized progesterone	100
	Progesterone vaginal suppository	25, 50
	Combinations	
Estratest	Esterified estrogen	1.25
	Methyltestosterone	2.5
Estratest HS	Esterified estrogen	0.625
	Methyltestosterone	1.25
Prempro	Conjugated estrogen	0.625
	Medroxyprogesterone acetate	2.5, 5
Premphase	Conjugated estrogen	0.625
	Medroxyprogesterone acetate	5
Activella	Estradiol	1.0
	Norethindrone acetate	0.5
FemHRT	Ethinyl estradiol	5 mcg
	Norethindrone acetate	1
CombiPatch	17 beta estradiol	0.05
	Norethindrone acetate	0.14, 0.25

Oral Contraceptives

- Consist of varying combinations of estrogen and progestin (combination pill), or progestin only ("minipill").
- Estrogens and progestins used in oral contraceptive preparations are listed in Table 9.3.
- The relative estrogenic, androgenic, and progestational activity of OC are listed in Table 9.4.
- Progestins produce both progestational and androgenic effects to varying degrees.
- Progestin-only pill ("minipill"):
  √ Includes Micronor (norethindrone), Ovrette (norgestrel)
  √ Advantages
    □ Since it lacks estrogen, can be used by women who should not use combined oral contraceptives (e.g., women with a history of blood clots and high blood pressure, or cigarette smokers over age of 35 years).
    □ Unlike combination pills, progestin-only pill does not diminish breast milk supply when used by nursing women.
  √ Disadvantages
    □ Less effective at preventing pregnancy (3–7% failure rate per year, in contrast to 0.5–1% with combination pill).
- In recent years, several new forms of contraception have become available that provide well-tolerated alternatives to the birth control pill. These include:
  √ Ortho-Evra (weekly contraceptive patch).
  √ NuvaRing (vaginal ring containing estrogen and progestin).
  √ Lea shield (diaphragm-like barrier).
  √ Mirena IUD (long-acting IUD coated with a progestin).
  √ Seasonale (daily oral contraceptive that limits menstruation to 1 week every 3 months).

Appendix 1
Drug Identification by Generic Name

Generic Name	Brand Name	Chief Action
alprazolam	Xanax	Anxiolytic
amantadine	Symmetrel	Antiparkinsonian, antiviral
amiloride	Mldamor	Potassium-sparing diuretic
amitriptyline	Elavil, Endep	Antidepressant
amoxapine	Asendin	Antidepressant
aripiprazole	Abilify	Antipsychotic
atenolol	Tenormin	Beta-blocker
atomoxetine	Strattera	Stimulant
benztropine	Cogentin	Antiparkinsonian anticholinergic
biperiden	Akineton	Antiparkinsonian anticholinergic
bromocriptine	Parlodel	Dopamine agonist
bupropion	Wellbutrin, Zyban	Antidepressant; also used for smoking cessation
buspirone	Buspar	Anxiolytic
cabergoline	Dostinex	Dopamine agonist
carbamazepine	Tegretol	Antiepileptic, mood stabilizer
chloral hydrate	Noctec	Hypnotic
chlorazepate	Tranxene	Anxiolytic
chlordiazepoxide	Librium	Anxiolytic
chlorpromazine	Thorazine	Antipsychotic
citalopram	Celexa, Lexapro (S-enantiomer)	Antidepressant
clomipramine	Anafranil	Antidepressant
clonazepam	Klonopin	Anxiolytic, antiepileptic
clozapine	Clozaril	Antipsychotic
desipramine	Norpramin, Pertofrane	Antidepressant
dextroamphetamine	Adderall, Dexedrine	Stimulant
diazepam	Valium	Anxiolytic
diethylpropion	Tenuate	Stimulant
divalproex	Depakote	Antiepileptic, mood stabilizer
donepezil	Aricept	Cholinergic function enhancer

(cont.)

Generic Name	Brand Name	Chief Action
(*cont.*)		
doxepin	Adapin, Sinequan	Antidepressant
droperidol	Inapsine	Antiemetic, anxiolytic, antipsychotic
duloxetine	Cymbalta	Antidepressant
estazolam	ProSom	Hypnotic
fluoxetine	Prozac, Sarafem	Antidepressant
fluphenazine	Prolixin, Permitil	Antipsychotic
flurazepam	Dalmane	Hypnotic
fluvoxamine	Luvox	Antidepressant
gabapentin	Neurontin	Antiepileptic, anxiolytic
halazepam	Paxipam	Anxiolytic
haloperidol	Haldol	Antipsychotic
hydroxyzine	Atarax, Vistaril	Antihistamine, anxiolytic
imipramine	Tofranil	Antidepressant
isocarboxazid	Marplan	Antidepressant
lamotrigine	Lamictal	Antiepileptic, mood stabilizer
levothyroxine	Synthroid	Thyroid hormone
liothyronine (T3)	Cytomel	Thyroid hormone
lithium	Eskalith, Lithane, Lithobid	Mood stabilizer
lorazepam	Ativan	Anxiolytic
loxapine	Loxitane	Antipsychotic
maprotiline	Ludiomil	Antidepressant
mesoridazine	Serentil	Antipsychotic
methamphetamine	Desoxyn	Stimulant
methylphenidate	Concerta, Focalin, Metadate, Methylin, Ritalin	Stimulant
methyltestosterone	Android	Androgen derivative
mirtazapine	Remeron	Antidepressant
modafinil	Provigil	Stimulant
molindone	Moban	Antipsychotic
naltrexone	ReVia	Narcotic antagonist
nefazodone	Serzone	Antidepressant
nortriptyline	Aventyl, Pamelor	Antidepressant
olanzapine	Zyprexa	Antipsychotic, antimanic agent
oxazepam	Serax	Anxiolytic
oxcarbazepine	Trileptal	Antiepileptic
paroxetine	Paxil	Antidepressant
pemoline	Cylert	Stimulant
perphenazine	Trilafon	Antipsychotic
phendimetrazine	Bontril, Plegine, Prelu-2	Stimulant
phenelzine	Nardil	Antidepressant
phentermine	Adipex, Fastin, Ionamin	Stimulant
pimozide	Orap	Antipsychotic
prazepam	Centrax	Anxiolytic
propranolol	Inderal	Beta-blocker
protriptyline	Vivactil	Antidepressant
quazepam	Doral	Hypnotic
quetiapine	Seroquel	Antipsychotic
quinagolide	Norprolac	Dopamine agonist

Generic Name	Brand Name	Chief Action
risperidone	Risperdal	Antipsychotic
selegiline	Eldepryl	Antidepressant
sertraline	Zoloft	Antidepressant
temazepam	Restoril	Hypnotic
thioridazine	Mellaril	Antipsychotic
thiothixene	Navane	Antipsychotic
topiramate	Topamax	Antiepileptic
tranylcypromine	Parnate	Antidepressant
trazodone	Desyrel	Antidepressant, hypnotic
triazolam	Halcion	Hypnotic
trifluoperazine	Stelazine	Antipsychotic
trihexyphenidyl	Artane	Antiparkinsonian, anticholinergic
trimipramine	Surmontil	Antidepressant
valproic acid	Depakene	Antiepileptic, mood stabilizer
venlafaxine	Effexor	Antidepressant
yohimbine	Yocon	Presynaptic alpha-2 antagonist
zaleplon	Sonata	Hypnotic
ziprasidone	Geodon	Antipsychotic
zolpidem	Ambien	Hypnotic

A
P
P
E
N
D
I
X

1

Appendix 2
Drug Identification by Brand Name

Brand Name	Generic Name	Chief Action
Abilify	aripiprazole	Antipsychotic
Adapin	doxepin	Antidepressant
Adderall	dextroamphetamine	Stimulant
Adipex	phentermine	Stimulant
Akineton	biperiden	Antiparkinsonian, anticholinergic
Ambien	zolpidem	Hypnotic, antiepileptic
Anafranil	clomipramine	Antidepressant
Android	methyltestosterone	Androgen derivative
Aricept	donepezil	Cholinergic function enhancer
Artane	trihexyphenidyl	Antiparkinsonian, anticholinergic
Asendin	amoxapine	Antidepressant
Atarax, Vistaril	hydroxyzine	Antihistamine, anxiolytic
Ativan	lorazepam	Anxiolytic
Aventyl	nortriptyline	Antidepressant
Benadryl	diphenhydramine	Antihistamine
Bontril	phendimetrazine	Stimulant
Buspar	buspirone	Anxiolytic
Celexa	citalopram	Antidepressant
Clozaril	clozapine	Antipsychotic
Cogentin	benztropine	Antiparkinsonian
Compazine	prochlorperazine	Antiemetic, dopamine blocker
Concerta	methylphenidate	Stimulant
Cylert	pemoline	Stimulant
Cymbalta	duloxetine	Antidepressant
Cytomel	liothyronine (T3)	Thyroid hormone
Dalmane	flurazepam	Hypnotic
Depakene	valproic acid	Antiepileptic, mood stabilizer
Depakote	divalproex	Antiepileptic, mood stabilizer
Desoxyn	d-methamphetamine	Stimulant
Desyrel	trazodone	Antidepressant

(cont.)

Brand Name	Generic Name	Chief Action
(cont.)		
Dexedrine	dextroamphetamine	Stimulant
Doral	quazepam	Hypnotic
Dostinex	cabergoline	Dopamine agonist
Effexor	venlafaxine	Antidepressant
Elavil	amitriptyline	Antidepressant
Eldepryl	selegiline	Antidepressant
Endep	amitriptyline	Antidepressant
Eskalith	lithium	Mood stabilizer
Fastin	phentermine	Sympathomimetic anorectic
Focalin	methyphenidate	Stimulant
Geodon	ziprasidone	Antipsychotic
Halcion	triazolam	Hypnotic
Haldol	haloperidol	Antipsychotic
Inapsine	droperidol	Antiemetic, anxiolytic, antipsychotic
Inderal	propanolol	Beta-blocker
Ionamin	phentermine	Sympathomimetic anorectic
Klonopin	clonazepam	Anxiolytic, antiepileptic
Lamictal	lamotrigine	Antiepileptic
Lexapro	s-citalopram	Antidepressant
Librium	chlordiazepoxide	Anxiolytic
Lithane	lithium	Mood stabilizer
Lithobid	lithium	Mood stabilizer
Loxitane	loxapine	Antipsychotic
Ludiomil	maprotiline	Antidepressant
Luvox	fluvoxamine	Antidepressant
Marplan	isocarboxazid	Antidepressant
Mellaril	thioridazine	Antipsychotic
Metadate	methyphenidate	Stimulant
Methylin	methyphenidate	Stimulant
Micronase	glyburide	Hypoglycemic
Midamor	amiloride	Potassium-sparing diuretic
Moban	molindone	Antipsychotic
Nardil	phenelzine	Antidepressant
Navane	thiothixene	Antipsychotic
Neurontin	gabapentin	Antiepileptic, anxiolytic
Noctec	chloral hydrate	Hypnotic
Norpramin	desipramine	Antidepressant
Norprolac	quinagolide	Dopamine agonist
Orap	pimozide	Antipsychotic
Pamelor	nortriptyline	Antidepressant
Parlodel	bromocriptine	Dopamine agonist
Parnate	tranylcypromine	Antidepressant
Paxil	paroxetine	Antidepressant
Paxipam	halazepam	Anxiolytic
Periactin	cyproheptadine	Antihistamine, serotonin antagonist
Permitil	fluphenazine	Antipsychotic
Pertofrane	desipramine	Antidepressant
Prelu-2	phendimetrazine	Stimulant
Preludin	phendimetrazine	Stimulant

Brand Name	Generic Name	Chief Action
Prolixin	fluphenazine	Antipsychotic
ProSom	estazolam	Hypnotic
Provigil	modafinil	Stimulant
Prozac	fluoxetine	Antidepressant
Remeron	mirtazapine	Antidepressant
Restoril	temazepam	Hypnotic
Risperdal	risperidone	Antipsychotic
Ritalin	methylphenidate	Stimulant
Sarafem	fluoxetine	Antidepressant
Seldane	terfenadine	Antihistamine
Serax	oxazepam	Anxiolytic
Serentil	mesoridazine	Antipsychotic
Seroquel	quetiapine	Antipsychotic
Serzone	nefazodone	Antidepressant
Sinequan	doxepin	Antidepressant
Sonata	zaleplon	Hypnotic
Stelazine	trifluoperazine	Antipsychotic
Strattera	atomoxetine	Stimulant
Surmontil	trimipramine	Antidepressant
Symmetrel	amantadine	Antiparkinsonian, antiviral
Synthroid	levothyroxine	Thyroid hormone
Tegretol	carbamazepine	Antiepileptic, mood stabilizer
Tenormin	atenolol	Beta-blocker
Tenuate	diethylpropion	Stimulant
Thorazine	chlorpromazine	Antipsychotic
Topamax	topiramate	Antiepileptic
Tranxene	clorazepate	Anxiolytic
Trilafon	perphenazine	Antipsychotic
Trileptal	oxcarbazepine	Antiepileptic
Valium	diazepam	Anxiolytic
Vistaril	hydroxyzine	Antihistamine, anxiolytic
Vivactil	protriptyline	Antidepressant
Wellbutrin	bupropion	Antidepressant
Xanax	alprazolam	Anxiolytic
Yocon	yohimbine	Presynaptic alpha-2 antagonist
Zoloft	sertraline	Antidepressant
Zyban	bupropion	Antidepressant; also used for smoking cessation
Zyprexa	olanzapine	Antipsychotic, mood stabilizer

A
P
P
E
N
D
I
X

2

GENERAL CONSIDERATIONS

American Academy of Pediatrics Committee on Drugs. The transfer of drugs and other chemicals into human milk. *Pediatrics.* 2001;108:776–789.

American Academy of Pediatrics Committee on Drugs. Use of psychoactive medication during pregnancy and possible effects on the fetus and newborn (RE9866). *Pediatrics.* 2000;105:880–887.

American Psychiatric Association. *Diagnostic and Statistical Manual of Mental Disorders* (4th ed.). Washington, DC: American Psychiatric Association, 1994.

Blazer DG. Psychiatry and the oldest old. *Am J Psychiatry.* 2000;157:1915–1924.

Burt VK, Suri R, Altshuler LL, Stowe ZN, Hendrick V, Muntean E. The use of psychotropic medications during breast-feeding. *Am J Psychiatry.* 2001;158:1001–1009.

Ensom MHH. Gender-based differences and menstrual cycle-related changes in specific diseases: Implications for pharmacotherapy. *Pharmacotherapy.* 2000;20:523–539.

Ernst CL, Goldberg JF. The reproductive safety profile of mood stabilizers, atypical antipsychotics, and broad-spectrum psychotropics. *J Clin Psychiatry.* 2002;63 Suppl 4:42–55.

Goodnick PJ, Chaudry T, Artadi J, Arcey S. Women's issues in mood disorders. *Expert Opin Pharmacother.* 2000;1:903–916.

Gopfert M, Webster J, Pollard Nelki. *Parental Psychiatric Disorder: Distressed Parents and Their Families.* Cambridge, U.K.: Cambridge University Press, 1996.

Hendrick V, Altshuler LL, Burt VK. Course of psychiatric disorders across the menstrual cycle. *Harv Rev Psychiatry.* 1996;4:200–207.

Hendrick V, Altshuler LL, Cohen L, Stowe Z. Evaluation of mental health and depression during pregnancy: Position paper. *Psychopharmacol Bull.* 1998;34:297–299.

Hendrick V, Burt VK, Altshuler LL. Psychotropic guidelines for breast-feeding mothers. *Am J Psychiatry.* 1996;153:1236–1237.

Kessler RC, McGonagle KA, Zhao S, et al. Lifetime and 12-month prevalence of *DSM-III-R* psychiatric disorders in the United States: Results from the National Comorbidity Survey. *Arch Gen Psychiatry.* 1994;51:8–19.

Masand PS. Weight gain associated with psychotropic drugs. *Expert Opin Pharmacother.* 2000;1:377–389.

Medical Economics Company. *Physicians' Desk Reference*, 55th Edition. Montvale, NJ:Author;2001.

Pollock BG. Gender differences in psychotropic drug metabolism. *Psychopharmacol Bull.* 1997;33:235–241.

Prout MN, Fish SS. Participation of women in clinical trials of drug therapies: A context for the controversies. *Medscape Women's Health Journal.* 2001;6(5):1.

Robinson GE. Women and psychopharmacology. *Medscape Women's Health eJournal.* 2002;7(1). Available at http://www.medscape.com/viewarticle/ 423938. Accessed September 4, 2003.

Roe CM, McNamara AM, Motheral BR. Gender- and age-related prescription drug use patterns. *Ann Pharmacother.* 2002;36:30–39.

Rosenthal NE, Sack DA, Gillin JC, et al. Seasonal affective disorder: A description of the syndrome and preliminary findings with light therapy. *Arch Gen Psychiatry.* 1984;41:72–80.

Roughan PA. Mental health and psychiatric disorders in older women. *Clin Geriatr Med.* 1993;9:173–190.

Simoni-Wastila L. Gender and psychotropic drug use. *Med Care.* 1998;36: 88–94.

GENDER DIFFERENCES IN PSYCHOPHARMACOLOGY

Abernethy DR, Greenblatt DJ, Divoll M, Arendt R, Ochs HR, Shader RI. Impairment of diazepam metabolism by low-dose estrogen-containing oral-contraceptive steroids. *N Engl J Med.* 1982;306:791–792.

Abernethy DR, Greenblatt DJ, Shader RI. Imipramine disposition in users of oral contraceptive steroids. *Clin Pharmacol Ther.* 1984;35:792–797.

Giles HG, Sellers EM, Naranjo CA, Frecker RC, Greenblatt DJ. Disposition of intravenous diazepam in young men and women. *Eur J Clin Pharmacol.* 1981;20:207–213.

Harris RZ, Benet LZ, Schwartz JB. Gender effects in pharmacokinetics and pharmacodynamics. *Drugs.* 1995;50:222–239.

Lane HY, Chang YC, Chang WH, Lin SK, Tseng YT, Jann MW. Effects of gender and age on plasma levels of clozapine and its metabolites: Analyzed by critical statistics. *J Clin Psychiatry.* 1999;60:36–40.

Pollock BG. Gender differences in psychotropic drug metabolism. *Psychopharmacol Bull.* 1997;33:235–241.

Sabers A, Buchholt JM, Uldall P, Hansen EL. Lamotrigine plasma levels reduced by oral contraceptives. *Epilepsy Res.* 2001;47:151–154.

Schatzberg AF, DeBattista C. Current psychotropic dosing and monitoring guidelines: 2002. *Primary Psychiatry.* 2002;9:34–48.

Stewart DE, Fairman M, Barbadoro S, Zownir P, Steiner M. Follicular and late luteal phase serum fluoxetine levels in women suffering from late luteal phase dysphoric disorder. *Biol Psychiatry.* 1994;36:201–202.

DEPRESSIVE DISORDERS

Ahokas A, Kaukoranta J, Wahlbeck K, Aito M. Estrogen deficiency in severe postpartum depression: Successful treatment with sublingual physiologic 17beta-estradiol—a preliminary study. *J. Clin Psychiatry.* 2001;62:332–336.

Altshuler LL, Hendrick V. Pregnancy and psychotropic medication: Changes in blood levels. *J Clin Psychopharmacol.* 1996;16:78–80.

Altshuler LL, Hendrick V, Cohen LS. Course of mood and anxiety disorders during pregnancy and the postpartum period. *J Clin Psychiatry.* 1998;59 Suppl 2:29–33.

American Psychiatric Association. *Practice Guidelines for the Treatment of Patients with; Major Depressive Disorder.* Washington, DC: American Psychiatric Press; 2000.

Amsterdam J, Garcia-Espana F, Fawcett J, Quitkin F, Reimherr F, Rosenbaum J, Beasley C. Fluoxetine efficacy in menopausal women with and without estrogen replacement. *J Affect Disord* 1999;55:11–17.

Appleby L, Warner R, Whitton A, Faragher B. A controlled study of fluoxetine and cognitive–behavioral counseling in the treatment of postnatal depression. *Br Med J.* 1997;314:932–936.

Aronson R, Offman HJ, Joffe RT, Naylor CD. Triiodothyronine augmentation in the treatment of refreactory depression. *Arch Gen Psychiatry.* 1996;53:842–848.

Avis NE, McKinlay SM. A longitudinal analysis of women's attitudes towards menopause: Results from the Massachusetts Women's Health Study. *Maturitas.* 1991;13:65–79.

Avis NE, McKinlay SM. The Massachusetts Women's Health Study: An epidemiologic investigation of the menopause. *JAMA.* 1995;50:45–49.

Baab SW, Peindl KS, Piontek CM, Wisner KL. Serum bupropion levels in 2 breastfeeding mother–infant pairs. *J Clin Psychiatry.* 2002;63:910–911.

Basson R, McInnes R, Smith MD, Hodgson G, Koppiker N. Efficacy and safety of sildenafil citrate in women with sexual dysfunction associated with female sexual arousal disorder. *J Womens Health Gend Based Med.* 2002;11:367–377.

Bauer M, Döpfemer S. Lithium augmentation in treatment-resistant depression: Meta-analysis of placebo-controlled studies. *J Clin Psychopharmacol.* 1999;19:427–434.

Bauer M, Whybrow PC. Thyroid hormone, neural tissue and mood modulation. *World J Biol Psychiatry.* 2001;2(2):59–69.

Birnbaum CS, Cohen LS, Bailey JW, Grush LR, Robertson LM, Stowe ZN. Serum concentrations of antidepressants and benzodiazepines in nursing infants: A case series. *Pediatrics.* 1999;104:e11.

Blacker, D. Maintenance treatment of major depression: A review of the literature. *Harv Rev Psychiatry.* 1996;4:1–9.

Brennan PA, Hammen C, Andersen MJ, Bor W, Najman JM, Williams GM. Chronicity, severity, and timing of maternal depressive symptoms: Relationships with child outcomes at age 5. *Dev Psychol.* 2000;36:759–766.

Briggs G, Freeman RK, Yaffe SJ, eds. *Drugs in Pregnancy and Lactation: A Reference Guide to Fetal and Neonatal risk* (5th ed.). Baltimore: Wilkins & Wilkins; 1998.

Burt VK, Altshuler LL, Rasgon N. Depressive symptoms in the perimenopause: Prevalence, assessment, and guidelines for treatment. *Harv Rev Psychiatry.* 1998;6:121–132.

Chambers CD, Anderson PO, Thomas RG, et al. Weight gain in infants breast-fed by mothers who take fluoxetine. *Pediatrics.* 1999;104:e61.

Chambers CD, Johnson KA, Dick BA, et al. Birth outcomes in pregnant women taking fluoxetine. *N Engl J Med.* 1996;335:1010–1015.

Chiu C, Huan S, Shen WW, Su K. Omega-3 fatty acids for depression in pregnancy. *Am J Psychiatry.* 2003;160(2):385.

Cohen LS, Heller VL, Bailey JW, Grush L, Ablon JS, Bouffard SM. Birth outcomes following prenatal exposure to fluoxetine. *Biol Psychiatry.* 2000;48:996–1000.

Cohen LS, Viguera AC, Bouffard SM, et al. Venlafaxine in the treatment of postpartum depression. *J Clin Psychiatry.* 2001;62:592–596.

Costei AM, Kozer E, Ho T, Ito S, Koren G. Perinatal outcome following third trimester exposure to paroxetine. *Arch Pediat Adolesc Med.* 2002;156:1129–1132.

Cox JL, Murray D, Chapman G. A controlled study of the onset, duration and prevalence of postnatal depression. *Br J Psychiatry.* 1993;163:27–31.

De Lima MS, Hotoph M, Wessely S. The efficacy of drug treatments for dysthymia: A systematic review and meta-analysis. *Psycholog Med.* 1999; 29:1273–1289.

DeVane CL. Pharmacogenetics and drug metabolism of newer antidepressant agents. *J Clin Psychiatry.* 1994;55(Suppl 12):38–45.

Diab T, Singh AN. The new generation of antidepressants. *Hosp Med.* 2003;64:12–15.

Einarson A, Fatoye B, Sarkar M, et al. Pregnancy outcome following gestational exposure to venlafaxine: A multicenter prospective controlled study. *Am J Psychiatry.* 2001;158:1728–1730.

Einarson A, Selby P, Koren G. Abrupt discontinuation of psychotropic drugs during pregnancy: Fear of teratogenic risk and impact of counseling. *J Psychiatry Neurosc.* 2001;26:44–48.

Entsuah AR, Huang H, Thase ME. Response and remission rates in different subpopulations with major depressive disorder administered venlafaxine, selective serotonin reuptake inhibitors, or placebo. *J Clin Psychiatry.* 2001;62:869–877.

Epperson CN, Anderson GM, McDougle CJ. Sertraline and breast-feeding. *N Engl J Med.* 1997;336:1189–1190.

Epperson N, Czarkowski KA, Ward-O'Brien D, et al. Maternal sertraline treatment and serotonin transport in breast-feeding mother–infant pairs. *Am J Psychiatry.* 2001;158:1631–1637.

Ericson A, Kullen B, Wilholm BE. Delivery outcome after the use of antidepressants in early pregnancy. *Eur J Clin Pharmacol.* 1999;55:503–508.

Fava, M. Management of nonresponse and intolerance: Switching strategies. *J Clin Psychiatry.* 2000;61(Suppl. 2):10–12.

Fava, M. New approaches to the treatment of refractory depression. *J Clin Psychiatry.* 2000;61(Suppl. 1):26–32.

Ferrill MJ, Kehoe WA, Jacisin JJ. ECT during pregnancy: Physiologic and pharmacologic considerations. *Convuls Ther.* 1992;8:186–200.

Frackiewicz EJ, Sramek JJ, Cutler NR. Gender differences in depression and antidepressant pharmacokinetics and adverse events. *Ann Pharmacother.* 2000;34:80–88.

Frank E, Kupfer DJ, Perel JM, et al. Three-year outcomes for maintenance therapies in recurrent depression. *Arch Gen Psychiatry.* 1990;47:1093–1099.

Frank E, Thase MF, Spanier CA, Reynolds CF, Kupfer DJ. Gender-specific response to depression treatment. *J Gend Specif Med.* 1999;2:40–44.

Fung MC. Olanzapine-exposed pregnancies and lactation: Early experience. *J Clin Psychopharmacol.* 2000;20:399–403.

Gardner DM, Shulman KI, Walker SE, Tailor SAN. The making of a user friendly MAOI diet. *J Clin Psychiatry.* 1996;57:99–104.

Gitlin MJ, Suri R. Management of side effects of SSRIs and newer antidepressants. In: R. Balon, ed. *Practical Management of the Side Effects of Psychotropic Drugs.* New York: Basel;1999:85–118.

Gold JH. Gender differences in psychiatric illness and treatments: A critical review. *J Nerv Ment Disord.* 1998;186:769–775.

Goldstein MZ. Depression and anxiety in older women. *Primary Care.* 2002;29:69–80.

Goodnick PJ, Chaudry T, Artadi J, Arcey S. Women's issues in mood disorders. *Expert Opin Pharmacother.* 2000;1:903–916.

Hammen C, Brennan PA. Severity, chronicity, and timing of maternal depression and risk for adolescent offspring diagnoses in a community sample. *Arch Gen Psychiatry.* 2003;60:253–258.

Harlow BL, Wise LA, Otto MW, Soares CN, Cohen LS. Depression and its influence on reproductive endocrine and menstrual cycle markers associated with perimenopause: The Harvard Study of Moods and Cycles. *Arch Gen Psychiatry.* 2003;60:29–36.

Hay DF, Pawlby S, Sharp D, Asten P, Mills A, Kumar R. Intellectual problems shown by 11-year-old children whose mothers had postnatal depression. *J Child Psychol Psychiatry.* 2001;42:871–889.

Hendrick V, Altshuler L. Management of major depression during pregnancy. *Am J Psychiatry.* 2002;159:1667–1673.

Hendrick V, Altshuler LL, Strouse T, et al. Postpartum and non-postpartum depression: Differences in presentation and response to pharmacologic treatment. *Depress Anxiety.* 2000;11:66–72.

Hendrick V, Altshuler L, Wertheimer A, Dunn WA. Venlafaxine and breast-feeding. *Am J Psychiatry.* 2001;158:2089–2090.

Hendrick V, Fukuchi A, Altshuler LL, et al. Use of sertraline, paroxetine and fluvoxamine by nursing women. *Brit J Psychiatry.* 2001;179:163–166.

Hendrick V, Smith LM, Suri R, Hwang S, Haynes D, Altshuler L. Birth outcomes after prenatal exposure to antidepressant medication. *Am J Obstet Gynecol.* 2003;188:812–815.

B
I
B
L
I
O
G
R
A
P
H
Y

Hirschfeld, RMA. Efficacy of SSRIs and newer antidepressants in severe depression: Comparison with TCAs. *J. Clin Psychiatry.* 1999;60:326–335.

Hostetter A, Stowe ZN, Strader JR Jr, McLaughlin E, Llewellyn A. Dose of selective serotonin uptake inhibitors across pregnancy: Clinical implications. *Depress Anxiety.* 2000;11:51–57.

Ilett KF, Hackett LP, Dusci LJ, et al. Distribution and excretion of venlafaxine and O-desmethylvenlafaxine in human milk. *Br J Clin Pharmacol.* 1998;45: 459–462.

Ilett KF, Kristensen JH, Hackett LP, Paech M, Kohan R, Rampono J. Distribution of venlafaxine and its O-desmethyl metabolite in human milk and their effects in breastfed infants. *Br J Clin Pharmacol.* 2002;53:17–22.

Kornstein SG. Gender differences in depression: Implications for treatment. *J Clin Psychiatry.* 1997;58:12–18.

Kornstein, SG, Schatzberg AF, Thase ME, et al. Gender differences in treatment response to sertraline versus imipramine in chronic depression. *Am J Psychiatry.* 2000;157:1445–1452.

Kornstein SG, Schatzberg AF, Thase ME, et al. Gender differences in chronic major and double depression. *J Affect Disord.* 2000;60:1–11.

Kristensen JH, Ilett KF, Hackett LP, et al. Distribution and excretion of fluoxetine and norfluoxetine in human milk. *Br J Clinical Pharmacol.* 1999;48:521–527.

Kulin NA, Pastuszak A, Sage SR, et al. Pregnancy outcome following maternal use of the new selective serotonin reuptake inhibitors: A prospective controlled multicenter study. *JAMA.* 1998;279:609–610.

Kumar C, McIvor RJ, Davies T, et al. Estrogen administration does not reduce the rate of recurrence of affective psychosis after childbirth. *J Clin Psychiatry.* 2003;64:112–118.

Laine K, Heikkinen T, Ekblad U, Kero P. Effects of exposure to selective serotonin reuptake inhibitors during pregnancy on serotonergic symptoms in newborns and cord blood monoamine and prolactin concentrations. *Arch Gen Psychiatry.* 2003;60:720–726.

Lawlor DA, Juni P, Ebrahim S, Egger M. Systematic review of the epidemiologic and trial evidence of an association between antidepressant medication and breast cancer. *J Clin Epidemiol.* 2003;56:155-163.

Lawrie TA, Herxheimer A, Dalton K. Oestrogens and progestogens for preventing and treating postnatal depression. *Cochrane Database Syst Rev.* 2000;(2):CD001690.

Lester BM, Cucca J, Andreozzi BA, et al. Possible association between fluoxetine hydrochloride and colic in an infant. *J Am Acad Child Adolesc Psychiatry.* 1993;32:1253–1255.

Lyons-Ruth K, Wolfe R, Lyubchik A, Steingard R. Depressive symptoms in parents of children under age three: Sociodemographic predictors, current correlates and associated parenting behaviors. In: Halfon N, Schuster M, Taaffe Young K, eds. *Child-Rearing in America: Challenges Facing Parents with Young Children.* New York: Cambridge University Press; 2002:217–262.

Martenyi F, Dossenbach M, Mraz K, Metcalfe S. Gender differences in the efficacy of fluoxetine and maprotiline in depressed patients: A double-blind trial of antidepressants with serotonergic or norepinephrinergic reuptake inhibition profile. *Eur Neuropsychopharmacol.* 2001;11:227–232.

McElhatton PR, Garebis HM, Eléfant E, et al. The outcome of pregnancy in 689 women exposed to therapeutic doses of antidepressants: A collaborative study of the European Network of Teratology Information Services (ENTIS). *Reprod Toxicol.* 1996;10:285–294.

Miller KJ, Conney JC, Rasgon NL, Fairbanks LA, Small GW. Mood symptoms and cognitive performance in women estrogen users and nonusers and men. *J Am Geriatr Soc.* 2002;50:1826–1830.

Miller LJ. Use of electroconvulsive therapy during pregnancy. *Hosp Commun Psychiatry.* 1994;45:444–450.

Murray L, Hipwell A, Hooper R, et al. The cognitive development of 5-year-old children of postnatally depressed mothers. *J Child Psychol Psychiatry.* 1996;37:927–933.

Nelson JC. Augmentation strategies in depression. *J Clin Psychiatry.* 2000; 61(Suppl. 2):13–19.

Nordeng H, Lindemann R, Perminov KV, et al. Neonatal withdrawal syndrome after in utero exposure to selective serotonin reuptake inhibitors. *Acta Paediatr.* 2001;90:288–291.

Nulman I, Rovet J, Stewart DE, et al. Neurodevelopment of children exposed in utero to antidepressant drugs. *N Engl J Med.* 1997;336:258–262.

Nulman I, Rovet J, Stewart DE, et al. Child development following exposure to tricyclic antidepressants or fluoxetine throughout fetal life: A prospective, controlled study. *Am J Psychiatry.* 2002;159:1889–1895.

O'Hara MW. *Postpartum Depression: Causes and Consequences.* New York: Springer-Verlag; 1995.

O'Hara MW, Swain AM. Rates and risk of postpartum depression—a meta-analysis. *Int Rev Psychiatry.* 1996;8:37–54.

Owens, MJ, Morgan, WN, Plott, SJ, Nemeroff, CB. Neurotransmitter receptor and transporter binding profile of antidepressants and their metabolites. *J Pharmacol Experiment Therapeutics.* 1997;283:1305–1322.

Pastuszak A, Schick-Boschetto B, Zuber C, Feldkamp M, Pinelli M, Sihn S, Donnenfeld A, McCormack M, Leen-Mitchell M, Woodland C, Gardner A, Hom M, Koren G. Pregnancy outcome following first-trimester exposure to fluoxetine (Prozac). *JAMA.* 1993;269:2246–2248.

Piccinelli M, Wilkinson G. Gender differences in depression: Critical review. *Br J Psychiatry.* 2000;177:486–492.

Pons G, Rey E, Matheson I. Excretion of psychoactive drugs into breast milk: Pharmacokinetic principles and recommendations. *Clin Pharmacokinet.* 1994;27:270–289.

Quitkin FM, Stewart JW, McGrath PJ, et al. Are there differences between women's and men's antidepressant responses? *Am J Psychiatry.* 2002;159:1848–1854.

Reiff-Eldridge R, Heffner CR, Ephross SA, Tennis PS, White AD, Andrews EB. Monitoring pregnancy outcomes after prenatal drug exposure through prospective pregnancy registries: A pharmaceutical company commitment. *Am J Obstet Gynecol.* 2000;182(1 Pt 1):159–163.

Reimherr FW, Amsterdam JD, Quitkin FM, et al. Optimal length of continuation therapy in depression: A prospective assessment during long-term fluoxetine treatment. *Am J Psychiatry.* 1998;155:1247–1253.

Rosenbaum JF, Fava M, Nierenberg AA, et al. Treatment-resistant mood disorders. In: Gabbard GO, ed. *Treatments of Psychiatric Disorders* (3rd ed.). Washington, DC: American Psychiatric Press; 2001:307–383.

Rubinow DR, Schmidt PJ, Roca C. Estrogen–serotonin interactions: Implications for affective regulation. *Biol Psychiatry.* 1998;44:839–850.

Sacheim HA, Prudic J, Devanand DP, et al. A prospective, randomized, double-blind comparison of bilateral and right unilateral electroconvulsive therapy at different stimulus intensities. *Arch Gen Psychiatry.* 2000;57:425–434.

Schmidt PJ, Nieman L, Danaceau MA, et al. Estrogen replacement in perimenopause-related depression: A preliminary report. *Am J Obstet Gynecol.* 2000;183:414–420.

Sherwin BB. Affective changes with estrogen and androgen replacement therapy in surgically menopausal women. *J Affect Disord.* 1988;14:177–187.

Simon GE, Cunningham ML, Davis RL. Outcomes of prenatal antidepressant exposure. *Am J Psychiatry.* 2002;159:2055–2061.

Soares CN, Almeida OP, Joffe H, Cohen LS. Efficacy of estradiol for the treatment of depressive disorders in perimenopausal women: A double-blind, randomized, placebo-controlled trial. *Arch Gen Psychiatry.* 2001;58:529–534.

Stewart DE, Boydell KM. Psychological distress during menopause: Associations across the reproductive life cycle. *Int J Psychiatry Med.* 1993;23:157–162.

Stone AB, Pearlstein TB: Evaluation and treatment of changes in mood, sleep and sexual functioning associated with menopause. *Obstet Gynecol Clin North Am.* 1994;1:391–403.

Stowe Z, Casarella J, Landry J, et al. Sertraline in the treatment of women with postpartum major depression. *Depression.* 1995;3:49–55.

Stowe ZN, Cohen LS, Hostetter A, et al. Paroxetine in human breast milk and nursing infants. *Am J Psychiatry.* 2000;157:185–189.

Stowe ZN, Owens MJ, Landry JC, et al. Sertraline and desmethylsertraline in human breast milk and nursing infants. *Am J Psychiatry.* 1997;154:1255–1260.

Suri R, Stowe ZN, Hendrick V, Hostetter A, Widawski M, Altshuler LL. Estimates of nursing infant daily dose of fluoxetine through breast milk. *Biol Psychiatry.* 2002;52:446–451.

Taddio A, Ito S, Koren G. Excretion of fluoxetine and its metabolite, norfluoxetine, in human breast milk. *J Clin Pharmacol.* 1996;36:42–47.

Wheeler Vega JA, Mortimer AM, Tyson PJ. Somatic treatment of psychotic depression: Review and recommendations for practice. *J Clin Psychopharmacol.* 2000;20:504–519.

Wisner KL, Gelenberg AJ, Leonard H, Zarin D, Frank E. Pharmacologic treatment of depression during pregnancy. *JAMA.* 1999;282:1264–1269.

Wisner KL, Perel JM, Peindl KS, et al. Prevention of recurrent postpartum depression. *J Clin Psychiatry.* 2001;62:82–86.

Wisner KL, Parry BL, Piontek CM. Postpartum depression. *N Engl J Med.* 2002;347;194–200.

Wisner KL, Perel JM, Blumer JF. Serum sertraline and N-desmethylsertraline levels in breast-feeding mother–infant pairs. *Am J Psychiatry.* 1998;155:690–692.

Yonkers KA, Brawman-Mintzer O. The pharmacologic treatment of depression: Is gender a critical factor? *J Clin Psychiatry.* 2002;63:610–615.

Young AH. Gender differences in treatment response to antidepressants. *Br J Psychiatry.* 2001;179:561.

BIPOLAR DISORDER

Adab N, Jacoby A, Smith D, et al. Additional educational needs in children born to mothers with epilepsy. *J Neurol Neurosurg Psychiatry.* 2001;70: 15–21.

Akiskal HS, Pinto O. The evolving bipolar spectrum: Prototypes I, II, III, and IV. *Psychiatr Clin North Am.* 1999;22:517–534.

American Psychiatric Association. *The Practice of Electroconvulsive Therapy: Recommendations for Treatment, Training, and Privileging—a Task Force Report of the American Psychiatric Association* (2nd ed.). Washington, DC: American Psychiatric Press; 2001.

Amsterdam JD, Garcia-Espana F. Venlafaxine monotherapy in women with bipolar II and unipolar major depression. *J Affect Disord.* 2000;59:225–229.

Bauer J, Isojarvi JI, Herzog AG, et al. Reproductive dysfunction in women with epilepsy: Recommendations for evaluation and management. *J Neurol Neurosurg Psychiatry.* 2002;73:121–125.

Blehar MC, DePaulo JR Jr, Gershon ES, Reich T, Simpson SG, Nurnberger JI Jr. Women with bipolar disorder: Findings from the NIMH Genetics Initiative sample. *Psychopharmacol Bull.* 1998;3:239–243.

Bowden CL, Brugger AM, Swann AC, et al. Efficacy of divalproex vs. lithium and placebo in the treatment of mania. *JAMA.* 1994;271:918–924.

Bowden CL, Calabrese JR, McElroy SL, et al. A randomized, placebo-controlled 12-month trial of divalproex and lithium in treatment of outpatients with bipolar I disorder. *Arch Gen Psychiatry.* 2000;57:481–489.

Calabrese JR, Bowden CL, Sachs GS, Ascher JA, Monaghan E, Rudd GD (Lamictal 602 Study Group). A double-blind placebo-controlled study of lamotrigine monotherapy in outpatients with bipolar I depression. *J Clin Psychiatry.* 1999;60:79–88.

Calabrese JR, Suppes T, Bowden CL, et al. A double-blind, placebo-controlled, prophylaxis study of lamotrigine in rapid-cycling bipolar disorder. *J Clin Psychiatry.* 2000;61:841–850.

Chaudron LH, Jefferson JW. Mood stabilizers during breastfeeding: A review. *J Clin Psychiatry.* 2000;61:79–90.

Cohen LS, Friedman JM, Jefferson JW, et al. A reevaluation of risk of in utero exposure to lithium. *JAMA,* 1994;271:146–150.

Compton MT, Nemeroff CB. The treatment of bipolar depression. *J Clin Psychiatry.* 2000;61 Suppl 9:57–67.

Coryell W, Keller M, Endicott J, Andreasen N, Clayton P, Hirschfield R. Bipolar II illness: Course and outcome over a five-year period. *Psycholog Med.* 1989;19:129–141.

Crawford P. Interactions between antiepileptic drugs and hormonal contraception. *CNS Drugs.* 2002;16:263–272.

De León OA. Antiepileptic drugs for the acute and maintenance treatment of bipolar disorder. *Harv Rev Psychiatry.* 2001;9:209–222.

Finnerty M, Levin Z, Miller LJ. Acute manic episodes in pregnancy. *Am J Psychiatry.* 1996;153:261–263.

Freeman MP, Smith KW, Freeman SA, McElroy SL, Kmetz GE, Wright R, Keck PE Jr. The impact of reproductive events on the course of bipolar disorder in women. *J Clin Psychiatry.* 2002;63:284–287.

Frey B, Schubiger G, Musy JP. Transient cholestatic hepatitis in a neonate associated with carbamazepine exposure during pregnancy and breast-feeding. *Eur J Pediatr.* 1990;150:136–138.

Frye MA, Ketter TA, Kimbrell TA, et al. A placebo-controlled study of lamotrigine and gabapentin monotherapy in refractory mood disorders. *J Clin Psychopharmacol.* 2000;20:607–614.

Gelenberg AJ, Kane JM, Keller MB, et al. Comparison of standard and low serum levels of lithium for maintenance treatment of bipolar disorder. *N Engl J Med.* 1989;321:1489–1493.

Gitlin M. Lithium and the kidney: An updated review. *Drug Safety.* 1999;20:231–243.

Goodwin FK, Jamison KR. *Manic–Depressive Illness.* New York: Oxford University Press; 1990.

Greil W, Ludwig-Mayerhofer W, Erazo N, et al. Lithium versus carbamazepine in the maintenance treatment of bipolar disorders—a randomized study. *J Affect Disord.* 1997;43:151–161.

Grof P, Robbins W, Alda M, et al. Protective effect of pregnancy in women with lithium-responsive bipolar disorder. *J Affect Disord.* 2000;61:31–39.

Hagg S, Spigset O. Anticonvulsant use during lactation. *Drug Safety.* 2000;22:425–440.

Hendrick V, Altshuler LL. Recurrent mood shifts of premenstrual dysphoric disorder can be mistaken for rapid-cycling bipolar II disorder. *J Clin Psychiatry.* 1998;59:479–480.

Hendrick V, Altshuler LL, Gitlin MJ, Delrahim S, Hammen C. Gender and bipolar illness. *J Clin Psychiatry.* 2000;61:393–396.

Hirschfeld RM, Allen MH, McEvoy JP, Keck PE Jr, Russell JM. Safety and tolerability of oral loading divalproex sodium in acutely manic bipolar patients. *J Clin Psychiatry.* 1999;60:815–818.

Iqbal MM, Gundlapalli SP, Ryan WG, Ryals T, Passman TE. Effects of antimanic mood stabilizing drugs on fetuses, neonates and nursing infants. *South Med J.* 2001;94:305–322.

Iqbal MM, Sohhan T, Mahmud SZ. The effects of lithium, valproic acid, and carbamazepine during pregnancy and lactation. *J Toxicol Clin Toxicol.* 2001;39:381–392.

Isojarvi JI, Tauboll E, Pakarinen AJ, et al. Altered ovarian function and cardiovascular risk factors in valproate-treated women. *Am J Med.* 2001;111:290–296.

Isojarvi JIT, Laatikainen TJ, Pakarinen AJ, et al. Polycystic ovaries and hyperandrogenism in women taking valproate for epilepsy. *N Engl J Med.* 1993;329:1383–1388.

Jacobson SJ, Jones K, Johnson X, et al. Prospective multicenter study of pregnancy outcome after lithium exposure during first trimester. *Lancet.* 1992;339:530–533.

Kallen B, Tandberg A. Lithium and pregnancy: A cohort study on manic–depressive women. *Acta Psychiatr Scand.* 1983;68:134–139.

Kleiner J, Altshuler L, Hendrick V, Hershman JM. Lithium-induced subclinical hypothyroidism: Review of the literature and guidelines for treatment. *J Clin Psychiatry.* 1999;60:249–255.

Kumar C, McIvor RJ, Davies T, et al. Estrogen administration does not reduce the rate of recurrence of affective psychosis after childbirth. *J Clin Psychiatry.* 2003;64:112–118.

La Marca A, Morgante G, Palumbo M, Cianci A, Petraglia F, De Leo V. Insulin-lowering treatment reduces aromatase activity in response to follicle-stimulating hormone in women with polycystic ovary syndrome. *Fertil Steril.* 2002;78:1234–1239.

Leibenluft E. Women and bipolar disorder: An update. *Bull Menninger Clin.* 2000;64:5–17.

Luef G, Abraham I, Haslinger M, et al. Polycystic ovaries, obesity and insulin resistance in women with epilepsy: A comparative study of carbamazepine and valproic acid in 105 women. *J Neurol.* 2002;249:835–841.

Matalon S, Schechtman S, Goldzweig G, Ornoy A. The teratogenic effect of carbamazepine: A meta-analysis of 1,255 exposures. *Reprod Toxicol.* 2002;16:9–17.

Merlob P, Mor M, Litwin A. Transient hepatic dysfunction in an infant of an epileptic mother treated with carbamazepine during pregnancy and breast-feeding. *Ann Pharmacother.* 1992;26:1563–1565.

Morrell MJ. The new antiepileptic drugs and women: Efficacy, reproductive health, pregnancy, and fetal outcome. *Epilepsia.* 1996;37 (Suppl 6):S34–44.

Morrell MJ. Epilepsy in women: The science of why it is special. *Neurology.* 1999;53(4 Suppl 1):S42–48.

Nemeroff CB, Evans DL, Gyulai L, et al. Double-blind, placebo-controlled comparison of imipramine and paroxetine in the treatment of bipolar depression. *Am J Psychiatry.* 2001;158:906–912.

Obrocea GV, Dunn RM, Frye MA, et al. Clinical predictors of response to lamotrigine and gabapentin monotherapy in refractory affective disorders. *Biol Psychiatry.* 2002;51:253–260.

O'Donovan C, Kusumakar V, Graves GR, Bird DC. Menstrual abnormalities and polycystic ovary syndrome in women taking valproate for bipolar mood disorder. *J Clin Psychiatry.* 2002;63:322–330.

Öhman I, Tomson T, Vitols S. Lamotrigine levels in plasma and breast milk in nursing women and their infants. *Epilepsia.* 1998;39(Suppl 2):21.

Öhman I, Vitols S, Luef G, Soderfeldt B, Tomson T. Topiramate kinetics during delivery, lactation, and in the neonate: Preliminary observations.: *Epilepsia.* 2002;43(10):1157–1160.

Öhman I, Vitols S, Tomson T. Lamotrigine in pregnancy: Pharmacokinetics during delivery, in the neonate, and during lactation. *Epilepsia.* 2000;41:709–713.

BIBLIOGRAPHY

Omtzigt JGC, Los FJ, Grobbee DE, et al. The risk of spina bifida aperta after first trimester exposure to valproate in a prenatal cohort. *Neurology.* 1992;42(Suppl 5):119–125.

Ornoy A, Cohen E. Outcome of children born to epileptic mothers treated with carbamazepine during pregnancy. *Arch Dis Child.* 1996;75:517–520.

Overpeck MD, Brenner RA, Trumble AC, Trifiletti LB, Berendes HW. Risk factors for infant homicide in the United States. *N Engl J Med.* 1998;339(1):211–216.

Pack AM, Morrell MJ. Adverse effects of antiepileptic drugs on bone structure: Epidemiology, mechanisms and therapeutic implications. *CNS Drugs.* 2001;15:633–642.

Pack AM, Morrell MJ. Treatment of women with epilepsy. *Semin Neurol.* 2002; 22:289–298.

Pfuhlmann B, Franzek E, Beckmann H, Stober G. Long-term course and outcome of severe postpartum psychiatric disorders. *Psychopathology.* 1999;32:192–202.

Pope HG Jr, McElroy SL, Keck PE Jr, Hudson JI. Valproate in the treatment of acute mania: A placebo-controlled study. *Arch Gen Psychiatry.* 1991;48: 62–68.

Rasgon NL, Altshuler LL, Gudeman D, et al. Medication status and polycystic ovary syndrome in women with bipolar disorder: A preliminary report. *J Clin Psychiatry.* 2000;61:173–178.

Robling SA, Paykel ES, Dunn VJ, Abbott R, Katona C. Long-term outcome of severe puerperal psychiatric illness: A 23 year follow-up study. *Psychol Med.* 2000;30:1263–1271.

Rosa FW. Spina bifida in infants of women treated with carbamazepine during pregnancy. *N Engl J Med.* 1991;324:674–677.

Small JG, Klapper MH, Kellams JJ, Miller MJ, Milstein V, Sharpley PH, Small IF. Electroconvulsive treatment compared with lithium in the management of manic states. *Arch Gen Psychiatry.* 1988;45:727–732.

Stahl MMS, Neiderud J, Vinge E. Thrombocytopenic purpura and anemia in a breast-fed infant whose mother was treated with valproic acid. *J Pediatrics.* 1997;130:1001–1003.

Stewart DE, Klompenhouwer JL, Kendell RE, van Hulst AM. Prophylactic lithium in puerperal psychosis: The experience of three centers. *Br J Psychiatry.* 1991;158:393–397.

Stoll AL, Severus WE, Freeman MP, et al. Omega 3 fatty acids in bipolar disorder: A preliminary double-blind, placebo-controlled trial. *Arch Gen Psychiatry.* 1999;56:407–412.

Suppes T, Webb A, Paul B, Carmody T, Kraemer H, Rush AJ. Clinical outcome in a randomized 1-year trial of clozapine versus treatment as usual for patients with treatment-resistant illness and a history of mania. *Am J Psychiatry.* 1999;156:1164–1169.

Tohen M, Sanger TM, McElroy SL, et al. Olanzapine versus placebo in the treatment of acute mania. *Am J Psychiatry.* 1999;156:702–709.

Tondo L, Baldessarini RJ. Rapid cycling in women and men with bipolar manic–depressive disorders. *Am J Psychiatry.* 1998;155:1434–1436.

Troyer WA, Perreira GR, Lannon RA, Belik J, Yoder MC. Association of maternal lithium exposure and premature delivery. *J Perinatology.* 1993;13:123–127.

Vasudev K, Goswami U, Kohli K. Carbamazepine and valproate monotherapy: Feasibility, relative safety and efficacy, and therapeutic drug monitoring in manic disorder. *Psychopharmacol* (Berlin). 2000;150:15–23.

Viguera AC, Cohen LS, Bouffard S, Whitfield TH, Baldessarini RJ. Reproductive decisions by women with bipolar disorder after prepregnancy psychiatric consultation. *Am J Psychiatry.* 2002;159:2102–2104.

Viguera AC, Nonacs R, Cohen LS, et al. Risk of recurrence of bipolar disorder in pregnant and nonpregnant women after discontinuing lithium maintenance. *Am J Psychiatry.* 2000;157:179–184.

Viguera AC, Tondo L, Baldessarini RJ. Sex differences in response to lithium treatment. *Am J Psychiatry.* 2000;157:1509–1511.

Wehr TA, Goodwin FK. Rapid cycling in manic depressives induced by tricyclic antidepressants. *Arch Gen Psychiatry.* 1979;36:555–559.

Yatham NY. The role of novel antipsychotics in bipolar disorders. *J Clin Psychiatry.* 2002;63(Suppl 3):10–14.

Yatham NY, Kusumakar V, Calabrese JR, Rao R, Scarrow G, Kroeker G. Third generation anticonvulsants in bipolar disorder: A review of efficacy and summary of clinical recommendations. *J Clin Psychiatry.* 2002;63:275–283.

Young LT, Joffe RT, Robb JC, MacQueen GM, Marriott M, Patelis-Siotis I. Double-blind comparison of addition of a second mood stabilizer versus an antidepressant to an initial mood stabilizer for treatment of patients with bipolar depression. *Am J Psychiatry.* 2000;157:124–126.

ANXIETY DISORDERS AND INSOMNIA

American Psychiatric Association. *Practice Guidelines for the Treatment of Patients with Panic Disorder.* Washington, DC: American Psychiatric Press;1998.

Bakker A, van Balkim AJLM, Spinhoven P. SSRIs vs. TCAs in the treatment of panic disorder: A meta-analysis. *Acta Psychiatr Scand.* 2002;106:163–167.

Blanco C, Antia SX, Liebowitz MR. Pharmacotherapy of social anxiety disorder. *Biol Psychiatry.* 2002;51:109–120.

Blier P, Bergeron R. Sequential administration of augmentation strategies in treatment-resistant obsessive–compulsive disorder: Preliminary findings. *Int Clin Psychopharmacol.* 1996;11:37–44.

Bogetto F, Venturello S, Albert U, Maina G, Ravizza L. Gender-related clinical differences in obsessive–compulsive disorder. *Eur Psychiatry.* 1999;14:434–441.

Bourdon KH, Boyd JH, Rae DS, et al. Gender differences in phobias: Results of the ECA community survey. *J Anx Disord.* 1988;2:227–241.

Breslau N. Gender differences in trauma and posttraumatic stress disorder. *J Gend Specif Med.* 2002;5:34–40.

Butterfield MI, Becker M, Marx CE. Post-traumatic stress disorder in women: current concepts and treatments. *Curr Psychiatry Rep.* 2002;4:474–486.

Dolovich LR, Addis A, Vaillancourt JM, Power JD, Koren G, Einarson TR. Benzodiazepine use in pregnancy and major malformations or oral cleft: Meta-analysis of cohort and case-control studies. *Br Med J.* 1998;317:839–843.

Fisher JB, Edgren BE, Mammel MC, Coleman JM. Neonatal apnea associated with maternal clonazepam therapy: A case report. *Obstet Gynecol.* 1985;88:345–355.

Foa EB, Davidson JRT, Frances A. The Expert Consensus Guidelines series: Treatment of posttraumatic stress disorder. *J Clin Psychiatry.* 1999;60(Suppl 16):1–76.

Gelpin E, Bonne O, Peri T, Brandes D, Shalev AY. Treatment of recent trauma survivors with benzodiazepines: A prospective study. *J Clin Psychiatry.* 1996;57:390–394.

Gorman JM. Treatment of generalized anxiety disorder. *J Clin Psychiatry.* 2002;63(Suppl 8):17–23.

Greist JH, Jefferson JW, Kobak KA, Katzelnik DJ, Serlin RC. Efficacy and tolerability of serotonin transport inhibitors in obsessive–compulsive disorder: A meta-analysis. *Arch Gen Psychiatry.* 1995;52:53–60.

Hageman I, Andersen HS, Jorgensen MB. Post-traumatic stress disorder: A review of psychobiology and pharmacotherapy. *Acta Pschiatr Scand.* 2001;104:411–422.

Hemmelgarn B, Suissa S, Huang A, et al. Benzodiazepine use and the risk of motor vehicle crash in the elderly. *JAMA.* 1997;278:27–31.

Hidalgo RB, Barnett SD, Davidson JRT. Social anxiety disorder in review: Two decades of progress. *Int J Neuropsychopharm.* 2001;4:279–298.

Hollander E, Bienstock CA, Koran LM, et al. Refractory obsessive–compulsive disorder: State-of-the-art treatment. *J Clin Psychiatry.* 2002;63(Suppl 6): 20–29.

Judd SJ, Wong J, Saloniklis S, et al. The effect of alprazolam on serum cortisol and luteinizing hormone pulsatility in normal women and in women with stress-related anovulation. *J Clin Endocrinol Metab.* 1995;80:818–823.

Kendler KS, Neale MC, Kessler RC, et al. Generalized anxiety disorder in women: A population-based twin study. *Arch Gen Psychiatry.* 1992;49:267–272.

Kendler KS, Neale MC, Kessler RC, et al. Panic disorder in women: A population-based twin study. *Psychol Med.* 1993;23:397–406.

McElhatton PR. The effects of benzodiazepine use during pregnancy and lactation. *Reprod Toxicol.* 1994;8:461–475.

McGrath C, Buist A, Norman TR. Treatment of anxiety during pregnancy: Effects of psychotropic drug treatment on the developing fetus. *Drug Safety.* 1999;20:171–186.

Montouris G. Gabapentin exposure in human pregnancy: Results from the Gabapentin Pregnancy Registry. *Epilepsy Behav.* 2003;4:310–317.

Ohayon MM. Prevalence of *DSM-IV* diagnostic criteria of insomnia: Distinguishing insomnia related to mental disorders from sleep disorders. *J Psychiatr Res.* 1997;31:333–346.

Ornoy A, Arnon J, Shechtman S, Moerman L, Lukashova I. Is benzodiazepine use during pregnancy really teratogenic? *Reprod Toxicol.* 1998;12:511–515.

Sandman CA, Wadhwa PD, Chickz-DeMet A, et al. Maternal stress, HPA activity and fetal/infant outcome. *Ann NY Acad Sci.* 1997;814:266–275.

Scheibe G, Albus M. Age at onset, precipitating events, sex distribution, and co-occurrence of anxiety disorders. *Psychopathology.* 1992;25:11–18.

Schneier FR. Treatment of social phobia with antidepressants. *J Clin Psychiatry.* 2001;62(Suppl 1):43–48.

Shader RI, Greenblatt DJ. Use of benzodiazepines in anxiety disorders. *N Engl J Med.* 1993;328:1398–1405.

Shear MK, Mammen O. Anxiety disorders in pregnant and postpartum women. *Psychopharmacol Bull.* 1995;31:693–703.

Sichel DA, Cohen LS, Dimmock JA, Rosenbaum JF. Postpartum obsessive-compulsive disorder: A case series. *J Clin Psychiatry.* 1993;54:156–159.

Van Ameringen M, Mancini C, Pipe B, Campbell M, Oakman J. Topiramate treatment for SSRI induced weight gain in anxiety disorders. *J Clin Psychiatry.* 2002;63:981–984.

Wadhwa PD, Sandman CA, Porto M, et al. The association between prenatal stress and infant birth weight and gestational age at birth: A prospective investigation. *Am J Obstet Gynecol.* 1993;169:858–865.

Walsh JK, Schweitzer PK. Ten-year trends in the pharmacological treatment of insomnia. *Sleep.* 1999;22:371–375.

Weinstock LS. Gender differences in the presentation and management of social anxiety disorder. *J Clin Psychiatry.* 1999;60(Suppl 9):9–13.

Whitelaw AGL, Cummings AJ, McFadden IR. Effect of maternal lorazepam on the neonate. *Br Med J.* 1981;282:1106–1108.

Yehuda R. Post-traumatic stress disorder. *N Engl J Med.* 2001;346:108–114.

Yonkers KA, Dyck IR, Keller MB. An eight-year longitudinal comparison of clinical course and characteristics of social phobia among men and women. *Psychiatr Services.* 2001;52:637–643.

SCHIZOPHRENIA

Adami HM, Verovsky IM, Thaker GK. Side effects of antipsychotic medications in women. *Primary Psychiatry.* 2002;9:50–54.

Adler LA, Rotrosen J, Edson R, et al. Vitamin E for tardive dyskinesia. *Arch Gen Psychiatry.* 1999;56:836–841.

Allison DB, Casey DE. Antipsychotic-induced weight gain: A review of the literature. *J Clin Psychiatry.* 2001;62(Suppl 7):22–31.

Almeida OP, Howard RJ, Levy R, David AS. Psychotic states arising in late life (late paraphrenia): The role of risk factors. *Br J Psychiatry.* 1995;166:215–228.

Alvir JM, Lieberman JA, Safferman AZ, Schwimmer JL, Schaaf JA. Clozapine-induced agranulocytosis: Incidence and risk factors in the United States. *N Engl J Med.* 1993;329:162–167.

American Psychiatric Association. Practice guidelines for the treatment of patients with schizophrenia. *Am J Psychiatry.* 1997;154(Suppl):1–63.

Azorin J-M, Spiegel R, Remington G, et al. A double-blind comparative study of clozapine and risperidone in the management of severe chronic schizophrenia. *Am J Psychiatry.* 2001;158:1305–1313.

Barnas C, Bergant A, Hummer M, Saria A, Fleishacker WW. Clozapine concentrations in maternal and fetal plasma, amniotic fluid, and breast milk. *Am J Psychiatry.* 1994;151:945.

Bottlender R, Jager M, Groll C, Strauss A, Moller HJ. Deficit states in schizophrenia and their association with the length of illness and gender. *Eur Arch Psychiatry Clin Neurosci.* 2001;251:272–278.

Canuso CM, Goldstein JM, Green AI. The evaluation of women with schizophrenia. *Psychopharmacol Bull.* 1998;34:271–277.

Casey DE. Tardive dyskinesia and atypical antipsychotic drugs. *Schizophr Res.* 1999;35 (Suppl):S61–S66.

Chakos M, Lieberman J, Hoffman E, et al. Effectiveness of second-generation antipsychotics in patients with treatment-resistant schizophrenia: A review and meta-analysis of randomized trials. *Am J Psychiatry.* 2001;158:518–526.

Collaborative Working Group on Clinical Trial Evaluations. Assessment of EPS and tardive dyskinesia in clinical trials. *J Clin Psychiatry.* 1998;59(Suppl 12):23–27.

Compton MT, Miller AH. Antipsychotic-induced hyperprolactinemia and sexual dysfunction. *Psychopharmacol Bull.* 2002;36:143–164.

Conley RR, Mahmoud R. A randomized double-blind study of risperidone and olanzapine in the treatment of schizophrenia or schizoaffective disorder. *Am J Psychiatry.* 2001;158:765–774.

Croke S, Buist A, Hackett LP, Ilett KF, Norman TR, Burrows GD. Olanzapine excretion in human breast milk: Estimation of infant exposure. *Neuropsychopharmacol.* 2002;5:243–247.

Csernansky JG, Mahmoud R, Brenner R. A comparison of risperidone and haloperidol for the prevention of relapse in patients with schizophrenia. *N Engl J Med.* 2002;346:16–22.

Dickson RA, Hogg L. Pregnancy of a patient treated with clozapine. *Psychiatric Services.* 1998;49:1081–1083.

Freeman MP. Omega-3 fatty acids in psychiatry: A review. *Ann Clin Psychiatry.* 2000;12:159–165.

Gardiner SJ, Kristensen JH, Begg EJ, et al. Transfer of olanzapine into breast milk, calculation of infant drug dose, and effect on breastfed infants. *Am J Psychiatry.* 2003;160:1428–1431.

Geddes J, Freemantle N, Harrison P, et al. Atypical antipsychotics in the treatment of schizophrenia: Systematic overview and meta-regression analysis. *Br Med J.* 2000;321:1371–1376.

Gilbert PL, Harris MJ, McAdams LA, et al. Neuroleptic withdrawal in schizophrenic patients: A review of the literature. *Arch Gen Psychiatry.* 1995;52:173–188.

Gitlin M, Nuechterlein K, Subotnik KL, et al. Clinical outcome following neuroleptic discontinuation in patients with remitted recent-onset schizophrenia. *Am J Psychiatry.* 2001;158:1835–1842.

Glassman AH, Bigger JT Jr. Antipsychotic drugs: Prolonged QTc interval, torsades de pointes, and sudden death. *Am J Psychiatry.* 2001;158:1774–1782.

Goff DC, Freudenreich O, Evins AE. Augmentation strategies in the treatment of schizophrenia. *CNS Spectrums.* 2001;6:904–911.

Goldstein DJ, Corbin LA, Fung MC. Olanzapine-exposed pregnancies and lactation: Early experience. *J Clin Psychopharm.* 2000;20:399–403.

Goldstein JM, Cohen LS, Horton NJ, Lee H, Andersen S, Tohen M, Crawford A, Tollefson G. Sex differences in clinical response to olanzapine compared with haloperidol. *Psychiatry Res.* 2002;110:27–37.

Goldstein JM, Link B. Gender and the expression of schizophrenia. *J Psychiatr Res.* 1988;22:141–155.

Goldstein JM, Seidman LJ, Goodman JM, Koren D, Lee H, Weintraub S, Tsuang MT. Are there sex differences in neuropsychological functions among patients with schizophrenia? *Am J Psychiatry.* 1998;155:1358–1364.

Harris RZ, Benet LZ, Schwartz JB. Gender effects in pharmacokinetics and pharmacodynamics. *Drugs.* 1995;50:222–239.

Hegarty JD, Baldessarini RJ, Tohen M, et al. One hundred years of schizophrenia: A meta-analysis of the outcome literature. *Am J Psychiatry.* 1994;151:1409–1416.

Howard LM, Goss C, Leese M, Thornicroft G. Medical outcome of pregnancy in women with psychotic disorders and their infants in the first year after birth. *Br J Psychiatry.* 2003;182:63–67.

Jeste DV, Caligiuri MP, Paulsen JS, et al. Risk of tardive dyskinesia in older patients: A prospective longitudinal study of 266 patients. *Arch Gen Psychiatry.* 1995;52:756–765.

Kane JM. Tardive dyskinesia in affective disorders. *J Clin Psychiatry.* 1999;60(Suppl 5):43–47.

Keck PE Jr, McElroy SL, Strakowski SM, Soutullo CA. Antipsychotics in the treatment of mood disorders and risk of tardive dyskinesia. *J Clin Psychiatry.* 2000;61(Suppl 4):33–38.

Kleinberg DL, Davis JM, de Coster R, et al. Prolactin levels and adverse events in patients treated with risperidone. *J Clin Psychopharmacol.* 1999;19:57–61.

Koren G, Cohn T, Chitayat D, Kapur B, Remington G, Reid DM, Zipursky RB. Use of atypical antipsychotics during pregnancy and the risk of neural tube defects in infants. *Am J Psychiatry.* 2002;159:136–137.

Koro CE, Fedder DO, L'Italien GJ, et al. An assessment of the independent effects of olanzapine and risperidone exposure on the risk of hyperlipidemia in schizophrenic patients. *Arch Gen Psychiatry.* 2002;59:1021–1026.

Kulkarni J, Riedel A, de Castella AR, Fitzgerald PB, Rolfe TJ, Taffe J, Burger H. Estrogen—a potential treatment for schizophrenia. *Schizophr Res.* 2001;48:137–144.

Lindamer LA, Buse DC, Lohr JB, Jeste DV. Hormone replacement therapy in postmenopausal women with schizophrenia: Positive effect on negative symptoms? *Biol Psychiatry.* 2001;49:47–51.

Lindamer LA, Lohr JB, Harris MJ, Jeste DV. Gender, estrogen, and schizophrenia. *Psychopharmacol Bull.* 1997;33:221–228.

Lindamer LA, Lohr JB, Harris J, McAdams LA, Jeste DV. Gender-related clinical differences in older patients with schizophrenia. *J Clin Psychiatry.* 1999;60:61–67.

Mah PM, Webster J. Hyperprolactinemia: Etiology, diagnosis, and management. *Semin Reprod Med.* 2002;20:365–374.

Melkersson KI, Hulting AL, Rane AJ. Dose requirements and prolactin elevation of antipsychotics in male and female patients with schizophrenia or related psychoses. *Br J Clin Pharmacol.* 2000;51:317–324.

Miyamoto S, Duncan GE, Goff DC, et al. Therapeutics of schizophrenia. In: KL Davis, D Charney, JT Coyle, C Nemeroff, eds. *Neuropsychopharmacology: The Fifth Generation of Progress.* Philadelphia: Lippincott, Williams & Wilkins; 2002:775–801.

Nicole L, Lesage A, Lalonde P. Lower incidence and increased male:female ratio in schizophrenia. *Br J Psychiatry.* 1992;161:556–557.

Nilsson E, Lichtenstein P, Cnattingius S, Murray RM, Hultman CM. Women with schizophrenia: Pregnancy outcome and infant death among their offspring. *Schizophr Res.* 2002;58:221–229.

Ratnayake T, Libretto SE. No complications with risperidone treatment before and throughout pregnancy and during the nursing period. *J Clin Psychiatry.* 2002;63(1):76–77.

Ryan MC, Collins P, Thakore JH. Impaired fasting glucose tolerance in first-episode, drug-naive patients with schizophrenia. *Am J Psychiatry.* 2003;160:284–289.

Seeman MV. The role of estrogen in schizophrenia. *J Psychiatry Neurosci.* 1996;21:123–127.

Seeman MV. Women and schizophrenia. *Medscape Women's Health eJournal.* 2000;5(2). Available at http://www.medscape.com/viewarticle/408915. Last accessed September 4, 2003.

Seeman MV. Women with schizophrenia as parents. *Primary Psychiatry.* 2002;9:39–42.

Slone D, Siskind V, Heinomen OP, et al. Antenatal exposure to the phenothiazines in relation to congenital malformations, perinatal mortality rate, birth weight and intelligence quotient score. *Am J Obstet Gynecol.* 1977;128:486–488.

Szymanski S, Lieberman JA, Alvir JM, et al. Gender differences in onset of illness, treatment response, course, and biologic indexes in first-episode schizophrenic patients. *Am J Psychiatry.* 1995;152:698–703.

Tamminga CA. Gender and schizophrenia. *J Clin Psychiatry.* 1997;58:33–37.

Taylor EA, Turner P. Anti-hypertensive therapy with propranolol during pregnancy and lactation. *Postgrad Med J.* 1981;57:427–430.

Trixler M, Tenyi T. Antipsychotic use in pregnancy: What are the best treatment options? *Drug Safety.* 1997;16:403–410.

Usall J, Araya S, Ochoa S, Busquets E, Gost A, Marquez M. Gender differences in a sample of schizophrenic outpatients. *Compr Psychiatry.* 2001;42:301–305.

Volavka J, Czobor P, Sheitman B, et al. Clozapine, olanzapine, risperidone, and haloperidol in the treatment of patients with chronic schizophrenia and schizoaffective disorder. *Am J Psychiatry.* 2002;159:255–262.

Wang PS, Walker AM, Tsuang MT, et al. Dopamine antagonists and the development of breast cancer. *Arch Gen Psychiatry.* 2002;59:1147–1154.

Wang PS, West JC, Tanielian T, et al. Recent patterns and predictors of antipsychotic medication regimens used to treat schizophrenia and other psychotic disorders. *Schizophr Bull.* 2000;26:451–457.

Winans EA. Antipsychotics and breastfeeding. *J Hum Lact.* 2001;17:344–347.

Wirshing DA, Spellberg BJ, Erhart SM, et al. Novel antipsychotics and new onset diabetes. *Biol Psychiatry*. 1998;44:778–783.

Woerner MG, Alvir JMJ, Saltz BL, et al. Prospective study of tardive dyskinesia in the elderly: Rates and risk factors. *Am J Psychiatry*. 1998;155:1521–1528.

Yoshida K, Smith B, Craggs M, Kumar R. Neuroleptic drugs in breast-milk: A study of pharmacokinetics and of possible adverse effects in breast-fed infants. *Psycholog Med*. 1998;28:81–91.

PMDD

Baker ER, Best RG, Manfredi RL, Demers LM, Wolf GC. Efficacy of progesterone vaginal suppositories in alleviation of nervous symptoms in patients with premenstrual syndrome. *J Assist Reprod Genet*. 1995;12:205–209.

Eriksson E, Andersch B, Ho HP, Landen M, Sundblad C. Diagnosis and treatment of premenstrual dysphoria. *J Clin Psychiatry*. 2002;63(Suppl 7):16–23.

Freeman EW. Evaluation of a unique oral contraceptive (Yasmin) in the management of premenstrual dysphoric disorder. *Eur J Contracept Reprod Health Care*. 2002;7(Suppl 3):27–34.

Freeman EW, Rickels K, Sondheimer SJ, Polansky M. A double-blind trial of oral progesterone, alprazolam, and placebo in treatment of severe premenstrual syndrome. *JAMA*. 1995;274:51–57.

Girman A, Lee R, Kligler B. An integrative medicine approach to premenstrual syndrome. *Am J Obstet Gynecol*. 2003;188(5 Suppl):S56–S65.

Grady-Weliky TA. Clinical practice: Premenstrual dysphoric disorder. *N Engl J Med*. 2003;348:433–438.

Halbreich U, Borenstein J, Pearlstein T, Kahn LS. The prevalence, impairment, impact, and burden of premenstrual dysphoric disorder (PMS/PMDD). *Psychoneuroendocrinology*. 2003;28(Suppl 3):1–23.

Jensvold MF, Reed K, Jarrett DB, et al. Menstrual cycle-related depressive symptoms treated with variable antidepressant dosage. *J Women's Health*. 1992;1:109–115.

Landen M, Eriksson E. How does premenstrual dysphoric disorder relate to depression and anxiety disorders? *Depress Anxiety*. 2003;17:122–129.

Ling FW. Recognizing and treating premenstrual dysphoric disorder in the obstetric, gynecologic, and primary care practices. *J Clin Psychiatry*. 2000;61(Suppl 12):9–16.

Sundstrom Poromaa I, Smith S, Gulinello M. GABA receptors, progesterone and premenstrual dysphoric disorder. *Arch Women Ment Health*. 2003;6:23–41.

Wyatt KM, Dimmock PW, O'Brien PM. Selective serotonin reuptake inhibitors for premenstrual syndrome. *Cochrane Database Syst Rev*. 2002;4:CD001396.

Wyatt K, Dimmock P, Jones P, Obhrai M, O'Brien S. Efficacy of progesterone and progestogens in management of premenstrual syndrome: Systematic review. *Br Med J*. 2001;323:776–780.

Yonkers K. Maintenance treatment of PMS: How long is long enough? *Archives of Women's Mental Health*. 2001;3(Suppl 2):8.

EATING DISORDERS

Appolinario JC, Fontenelle LF, Papelbaum M, Bueno JR, Coutinho W. Topiramate use in obese patients with binge eating disorder: An open study. *Can J Psychiatry.* 2002;47:271–273.

Appolinario JC, Godoy-Matos A, Fontenelle LF, et al. An open-label trial of sibutramine in obese patients with binge-eating disorder. *J Clin Psychiatry.* 2002;63:28–30.

Arnold LM, McElroy SL, Hudson JI, Welge JA, Bennett AJ, Keck PE. A placebo-controlled, randomized trial of fluoxetine in the treatment of binge-eating disorder. *J Clin Psychiatry.* 2002;63:1028–1033.

Becker AE, Grinspoon SK, Klibanski A, Herzog DB. Eating disorders. *N Engl J Med.* 1999;340;1092–1098.

Casper RC. Recognizing eating disorders in women. *Psychopharmacol Bull.* 1998;34:267–269.

Casper RC. How useful are pharmacological treatments in eating disorders? *Psychopharmacol Bull.* 2002 S;36:88–104.

Dingemans AE, Bruna MJ, van Furth EF. Binge eating disorder: A review. *Int J Obes Relat Metab Disord.* 2002;26:299–307.

Franko DL, Blais MA, Becker AE, et al. Pregnancy complications and neonatal outcomes in women with eating disorders. *Am J Psychiatry.* 2001;158:1461–1466.

Franko DL, Spurrell EB. Detection and management of eating disorders during pregnancy. *Obstet Gynecol.* 2000;95(6 Pt 1):942–946.

Goldbloom DS. Pharmacotherapy of bulimia nervosa. *Medscape Women's Health.* 1997;2:4.

Herzog DB, Greenwood DN, Dorer DJ, et al. Mortality in eating disorders: A descriptive study. *Int J Eat Disord.* 2000;28:20–26.

James DC. Eating disorders, fertility, and pregnancy: Relationships and complications. *J Perinat Neonatal Nurs.* 2001;15:36–48.

Keel PK, Mitchell JE, Miller KB, Davis TI, Crow SJ. Long-term outcome of bulimia nervosa. *Arch Gen Psychiatry.* 1999;56:63–69.

Kennedy SH, Piran N, Warsh JJ, et al. A trial of isocarboxazid in the treatment of bulimia nervosa. *J Clin Psychopharmacol.* 1988;8:391–396.

Kinzl JF, Traweger C, Trefalt E, Mangweth B, Biebl W. Binge eating disorder in females: A population-based investigation. *Int J Eat Disord.* 1999;25:287–292.

Mayer LE, Walsh BT. The use of selective serotonin reuptake inhibitors in eating disorders. *J Clin Psychiatry.* 1998;59(Suppl 15):28–34.

McElroy SL, Arnold LM, Shapira NA, et al. Topiramate in the treatment of binge eating disorder associated with obesity: A randomized, placebo-controlled trial. *Am J Psychiatry.* 2003;160:255–261.

Mitchell JE, Peterson CB, Myers T, Wonderlich S. Combining pharmacotherapy and psychotherapy in the treatment of patients with eating disorders. *Psychiatr Clin North Am.* 2001;24:315–323.

Morgan JF, Lacey JH, Sedgwick PM. Impact of pregnancy on bulimia nervosa. *Br J Psychiatry.* 1999;174:135–140.

Morrill ES, Nickols-Richardson HM. Bulimia nervosa during pregnancy: A review. *J Am Diet Assoc.* 2001;101:448–454.

Nakash-Eisikovits O, Dierberger A, Westen D. A multidimensional meta-analysis of pharmacotherapy for bulimia nervosa: Summarizing the range of outcomes in controlled clinical trials. *Harv Rev Psychiatry.* 2002;10:193–211.

Powers PS, Santana CA. Eating disorders: A guide for the primary care physician. *Primary Care.* 2002;29:81–98.

Ricca V, Mannucci E, Mezzani B, et al. Fluoxetine and fluvoxamine combined with individual cognitive–behavior therapy in binge eating disorder: A one-year follow-up study. *Psychother Psychosom.* 2001;70:298–306.

Romano SJ, Halmi KA, Sarkar NP, Koke SC, Lee JS. A placebo-controlled study of fluoxetine in continued treatment of bulimia nervosa after successful acute fluoxetine treatment. *Am J Psychiatry.* 2002;159:96–102.

Rosenblum J, Forman S. Evidence-based treatment of eating disorders. *Curr Opin Pediatr.* 2002;14:379–383.

Schmidt do Prado-Lima PA, Bacaltchuck J. Topiramate in treatment-resistant depression and binge-eating disorder. *Bipolar Disord.* 2002;4:271–273.

Stein A, Fairburn CG. Eating habits and attitudes in the postpartum period. *Psychosom Med.* 1996;58:321–325.

Steinhausen HC. The outcome of anorexia nervosa in the 20th century. *Am J Psychiatry.* 2002;159:1284–1293.

Vitiello B, Lederhendler I. Research on eating disorders: Current status and future prospects. *Biol Psychiatry.* 2000;47:777–786.

Westen D, Harnden-Fischer J. Personality profiles in eating disorders: Rethinking the distinction between Axis I and Axis II. *Am J Psychiatry.* 2001;158:547–562.

Wilson GT, Fairburn CG. Treatments for eating disorders. In: Nathan PE, Gorman JM, eds. *A Guide to Treatments That Work* (2nd ed.). New York: Oxford University Press; 2002:559–592.

Zerbe KJ. Medical complications of eating disorders. Available at http://cyberounds.com/conferences/psychiatry/conferences/0900/index.html. Last accessed September 4, 2003.

FEMALE REPRODUCTIVE HORMONES AND THE CENTRAL NERVOUS SYSTEM

Amsterdam J, Garcia-Espana F, Fawcett J, et al. Fluoxetine efficacy in menopausal women with and without estrogen replacement. *J Affect Disord.* 1999;55:11–17.

Bancroft J, Sanders D, Warner P, et al. The effects of oral contraceptives on mood and sexuality: A comparison of triphasic and combined preparations. *J Psychosom Obstetr Gynecol.* 1987;7:1–8.

Birkhauser M. Depression, menopause and estrogens: Is there a correlation? *Maturitas.* 2002;41 Suppl 1:S3–S8.

Burkman RT. Oral contraceptives: Current status. *Clin Obstet Gynecol.* 2001;44:62–72.

Davis SR, Tran J. Testosterone influences libido and well-being in women. *Trends Endocrinol Metab.* 2001;12:33–37.

Epperson CN, Wisner KL, Yamamoto B. Gonadal steroids in the treatment of mood disorders. *Psychosom Med.* 1999;61:676–697.

Fink G, Sumner BE, McQueen JK, Wilson H, Rosie R. Sex steroid control of mood, mental state and memory. *Clin Exp Pharmacol Physiol.* 1998;25:764–775.

Gonzales GF, Carrillo C. Blood serotonin levels in postmenopausal women: Effects of age and serum oestradiol levels. *Maturitas.* 1993;17:23–29.

Graham CA, Sherwin BB. The relationship between mood and sexuality in women using an oral contraceptive as a treatment for premenstrual symptoms. *Psychoneuroendocrinol.* 1993;18:273–281.

Grigoriadis S, Kennedy SH. Role of estrogen in the treatment of depression. *Am J Ther.* 2002;9:503–509.

Grimes DA, Lobo RA. Perspectives on the Women's Health Initiative trial of hormone replacement therapy. *Obstet Gynecol.* 2002;100:1344–1353.

Kaunitz AM. Long-acting hormonal contraception: Assessing impact on bone density, weight, and mood. *Int J Fertil Womens Med.* 1999;44:110–117.

Klaiber EL, Broverman DM, Vogel W, Peterson LG, Snyder MB. Relationships of serum estradiol levels, menopausal duration, and mood during hormonal replacement therapy. *Psychoneuroendocrinol.* 1997;22:549–558.

Kolsch H, Rao ML. Neuroprotective effects of estradiol-17beta: Implications for psychiatric disorders. *Arch Women Ment Health.* 2002;5:105–110.

Mishell Dr Jr, Darney PD, Burkman RT, Sulak PJ. Practice guidelines for OC selection: Update. *Dialogues Contracept.* 1997;5:7–20.

Nelson HD, Humphrey LL, Nygren P, Teutsch SM, Allan JD. Postmenopausal hormone replacement therapy: Scientific review. *JAMA.* 2002;288: 872–881.

Oinonen KA, Mazmanian D. To what extent do oral contraceptives influence mood and affect? *J Affect Disord.* 2002;70:229–240.

Pearce MJ, Hawton K. Psychological and sexual aspects of the menopause and HRT. *Baillieres Clin Obstet Gynaecol.* 1996;10:385–399.

Riecher-Rossler A. Oestrogen effects in schizophrenia and their potential therapeutic implications—review. *Arch Women Ment Health.* 2002;5:111–118.

Rubinow DR, Schmidt PJ, Roca C. Estrogen–serotonin interactions: Implications for affective regulation. *Biol Psychiatry.* 1998;44:839–850.

Schechter D. Estrogen, progesterone, and mood. *J Gend Specif Med.* 1999;2:29–36.

Schmidt PJ, Nieman L, Danaceau MA, et al. Estrogen replacement in perimenopause-related depression: A preliminary report. *Am J Obstet Gynecol.* 2000;183:414–420.

Sherwin BB. Affective changes with estrogen and androgen replacement therapy in surgically menopausal women. *J Affect Disord.* 1988;14:177–187.

Sherwin BB, Gelfand MM, Brender W. Androgen enhances sexual motivation in females: A prospective, crossover study of sex steroid administration in the surgical menopause. *Psychosom Med.* 1985;47:339–351.

Soares CN, Almeida OP, Joffe H, Cohen LS. Efficacy of estradiol for the treatment of depressive disorders in perimenopausal women: A double-blind, randomized, placebo-controlled trial. *Arch Gen Psychiatry.* 2001;58:529–534.

Soares CN, Poitras JR, Prouty J. Effect of reproductive hormones and selective estrogen receptor modulators on mood during menopause. *Drugs Aging.* 2003;20:85–100.

Stahl SM. Natural estrogen as an antidepressant for women. *J Clin Psychiatry.* 2001;62:404–405.

Stoppe G, Doren M. Critical appraisal of effects of estrogen replacement therapy on symptoms of depressed mood. *Arch Women Ment Health.* 2002;5:39–47.

Teichmann AT. Influence of oral contraceptives on drug therapy. *Am J Obstet Gynecol.* 1990;163(6 Pt 2):2208–2213.

Warnock JK, Bundren JC, Morris DW. Depressive symptoms associated with gonadotropin-releasing hormone agonists. *Depress Anxiety.* 1998;7:171–177.

Westhoff C, Wieland D, Tiezzi L. Depression in users of depomedroxyprogesterone acetate. *Contraception.* 1995;51:351–354.

Yen SSC, Jaffe RB, Barbieri RL. *Reproductive Endocrinology: Physiology, Pathophysiology and Clinical Management* (4th Ed.). Philadelphia: WB Saunders; 1999.

Yonkers KA, Bradshaw KD. Hormone replacement and oral contraceptive therapy: Do they induce or treat mood symptoms? In: Leibenluft E, ed. *Gender Differences in Mood and Anxiety Disorders.* Washington, DC: American Psychiatric Press; 1999: 91–135.

Young EA, Korszun A. The hypothalamic–pituitary–gonadal axis in mood disorders. *Endocrinol Metab Clin North Am.* 2002;31:63–78.

WEBSITES

www.anred.com
Depression After Delivery at: *www.depressionafterdelivery.com*
www.fda.gov/womens/registries/learnmore/html
www.4woman.gov
www.labcorp.com/datasets/labcorp/html/chapter/index.htm
www.motherisk.org
www.nida.nih.gov/WHGD/WHGDHome.html
www.nimh.nih.gov/wmhc/index.cfm
www.otispregnancy.org
Postpartum Support International at: *www.postpartum.net*
www.womens-health.com
www.womensmentalhealth.org

Index

I
N
D
E
X

INDEX